Dyslexia

Dyslexia
Interdisciplinary Approaches to Reading Disabilities

Herman K. Goldberg, M.D.
Chief of Ophthalmology
Sinai Hospital of Baltimore
Associate Professor of Ophthalmology and
Associate Professor of Pediatrics
The Johns Hopkins School of Medicine
Baltimore, Maryland

Gilbert B. Schiffman, Ed.D.
Coordinator of Exceptional Children Programs and
Professor of Education
The Johns Hopkins University
Assistant Professor of Education
Department of Pediatrics
The Johns Hopkins School of Medicine
Senior Consultant in Education
The John F. Kennedy Institute for Handicapped Children
Baltimore, Maryland

Michael Bender, Ed.D.
Director of Special Education
The John F. Kennedy Institute for Handicapped Children
Associate Professor of Education
The Johns Hopkins University
Assistant Professor of Special Education
Department of Pediatrics
The Johns Hopkins School of Medicine
Baltimore, Maryland

With a foreword by
Leo Kanner, M.D.
Professor Emeritus of Child Psychiatry and Honorary Consultant
The John Hopkins School of Medicine
Baltimore, Maryland

 Grune & Stratton
A Subsidiary of Harcourt Brace Jovanovich, Publishers
New York   London
Paris   San Diego   San Francisco
São Paulo   Sydney   Tokyo   Toronto

Library of Congress Cataloging in Publication Data
Main entry under title:

Dyslexia, interdisciplinary approaches to reading
    disabilities.

    Bibliography
    Includes index.
        1. Dyslexia.   2.Reading disability.   I. Goldberg,
Herman K.   II. Schiffman, Gilbert B.   III. Bender
Michael, 1943–
RJ496.A5D97   1983   616.85′53   82-15824
ISBN 0-8089-1484-7

Grune & Stratton, Inc.
111 Fifth Avenue
New York, New York 10003

Distributed in the United Kingdom by
Academic Press Inc. (London) Ltd.
24/28 Oval Road, London NW 1

Library of Congress Catalog Number 82-15824
International Standard Book Number 0-8089-1484-7

Printed in the United States of America

To Dolly, for her patience and enduring support.

To "A," without whose support the world would have no meaning.

To Joan, Al, Andrew, Scott, and Amy, with all my love.

To Leo Kanner, 1884–1981, a great teacher, physician, and friend, whose influence will be greatly missed.

Contents

Acknowledgments

We would like to express our sincere appreciation for the assistance offered by many of our staff and colleagues during the writing of this edition. Without their support this arduous task would not have been completed.

We are most grateful to Kevin Dwyer, M.A., a psychologist in the Montgomery County public school system, Montgomery County, Maryland, for his insight and efforts in writing the chapter entitled, "Psychological Evaluation" (Chapter 3). His clinical expertise and suggestions were welcomed, timely, and relevant.

We thank Marcia Pearce Burgdorf, J.D., President of the Developmental Disabilities Law Project, Inc., Baltimore, Maryland, and Assistant Professor, University of Maryland School of Law, for insightful comments on the chapters involving legal considerations (Chapters 13 and 14).

We recognize Dr. Brad W. Friedrich, Chief of Audiology at the John F. Kennedy Insitute in Baltimore, Maryland, who assisted in reviewing, editing, and re-reviewing the chapter, "Hearing and Auditory Perception" (Chapter 8). Dr. Friedrich's recommendations have provided the authors with much information and insight into the hearing and auditory processes of learning disabled children.

A special acknowledgment is extended to Dr. M. E. B. Lewis, Principal of the The John F. Kennedy Learning Disability School, Baltimore, Maryland, who undertook the most difficult and time-consuming task of reviewing and editing the entire manuscript. Dr. Lewis' countless hours in meeting with the authors and providing continual suggestions was much appreciated.

A special thank you is offered to Mr. Zanvyl Kreiger, who continously provided research support and assistance for many of the author's efforts, and to Lorraine Richter, Shirley Justice, and Eileen Lesser for their typing, retyping, editing, and patience in preparing this manuscript.

Foreword

In this era of unprecented publication explosion there is hardly a topic in any area of human interest that has not been seized upon by the printing press. Articles by the tens of thousands and monographs and books by the countless dozens are foisted on the reading public in an unending flow brought out in scientific and lay journals, in volumes by single authors, and in symposia and edited tomes with a host of contributors.

The problem of dyslexia, more commonly referred to as specific learning disability of reading, did not fail to share this fate. This issue, virtually unknown to the general public before Hinshelwood brought out his book on congenital word blindness (1900), has resulted in an astronomical effusion which, if assembled together, could easily fill many shelves of a large special library. There has been an avalanche of varieties of nomenclature, etiological theories, therapeutic "thou-shalts" and "thou-shalt-nots," serious research studies, good-will sermons, and just plain verbiage.

As one who has lived through this development from its beginning, I have witnessed pontifical assertions of a genetic origin, pseudoneurological edicts about conflict of cerebral dominance, pseudodynamic reference to psychoanalytic principles, and variegated educational groping.

This is not to say that important work has not been done and reported. Concerned people in the fields of education, neurology, psychology, psychiatry, and ophthalmology have done their best to become acquainted with the study, understanding, and remedy of the difficulty and its ramifications. However, there has been a remarkable dearth of intercommunication so that we are still confronted with the spectacle of the different disciplines working in isolation, sometimes finding themselves somnambulating in each others' camps.

---

*Hinshelwood, J. Congenital word blindness. *Lancet,* 1900, *1:* 1506–1508

For this reason it is refreshing to come upon a valiant effort that pulls together all the factual knowledge obtained thus far and that integrates the various fragments into a substantial edifice centering on the one thing that is common to all the building stones, namely, the individual child who is the victim of the difficulty and who needs primary consideration.

Dr. Herman K. Goldberg, an outstanding ophthalmologist who has given earnest attention to children and their reading disabilities, has made himself thoroughly familiar with all the aspects of the reading disability problem. He has done so with an astute ability to extract the scientifically established facts without espousing any unproven hypothesis and tradition and has coordinated solid, indisputable data from the areas of early predictability, psychology and psychological evaluation, neurological considerations, visual and auditory factors, psychiatric implications, and biochemical investigations. Such an undertaking has been long overdue. While this manner of presentation accentuates the complexity of the problem, it nevertheless works at the same time toward a welcome clarification.

Dr. Goldberg, who in his medical setting has not had any direct teaching experience with learning disabled children, has had the profound wisdom to invite and receive the collaboration of Dr. Gilbert B. Schiffman, a nationally prominent educator who, as part of his universal pedagogic interests, has given a great deal of attention to the problems of reading disabilities. He is the author of the chapters entitled, "The Scope of the Reading Problem" and "The Evaluation and Instruction of the Severely Disabled Reader," in which his authoritative familiarity with reading disabilities rings through every sentence.

In this edition, Dr. Goldberg and Dr. Schiffman have appropriately requested that Dr. Michael Bender, an international authority in the area of the handicapped child and a well-known advocate for the handicapped and their parents, participate in the authorship of this book so that parents, physicians, and educators can be made aware of the child's rights as provided by current federal legislation. Dr. Bender emphasizes the need for each child to have the right to an appropriate education in the least restrictive environment.

This edition can be of considerable use to those concerned with children's reading, be they educators, psychiatrists, psychologists, pediatricians, family physicians, ophthalmologists, or sufficiently educated parents.

Having had four decades of contact with children and their many problems, I can say that I have enjoyed reading this book and have profited from it.

LEO KANNER, M.D.
*Professor Emeritus of Child Psychiatry
and Honorary Consultant
The Johns Hopkins School of Medicine
Baltimore, Maryland*

Dyslexia

1

Overview of the Reading Disability Problem

This book is a revised edition of *Dyslexia: Problems of Reading Disabilities* (Goldberg and Schiffman, 1972). Since then, there have been major changes in educational practices and legal mandates that directly affect individuals with severe reading problems. The most significant legislation passed since the original publication was Public Law 94-142, the "Education of All Handicapped Children Act."* Specifically, it is the purpose of this act to

... assure that all handicapped children have available to them. ... a free appropriate public education which emphasizes special education and related services designed to meet their unique needs, to assure that the rights of handicapped children and their parents or guardians are protected, to assist states and localities to provide for the education of all handicapped children, and to assess and assure the effectiveness of efforts to educate handicapped children (PL 94-142).

The reader will notice that the term "learning disability" is now used in this revised edition as well as the word "dyslexia." This is due in part to the more general acceptance of the former term as a description of children with complex learning problems including severe reading delay. By federal definition a learning disability is

---

*While there are recently some moves to reassess the federal commitment to the handicapped, state and local education agencies continue to implement this mandate.

A disorder in one of more of the basic psychological processes involved in understanding or in using language, spoken or written, which may manifest itself in an imperfect ability to listen, think, speak, read, write, spell, or to do mathematical calculations. The term includes such conditions as perceptual handicaps, brain injury, minimal brain dysfunction, dyslexia, and development aphasia. The term does not include children who have learning problems which are primarily the result of visual, hearing, or motor handicaps, of mental retardation, or of environmental, cultural, or economic disadvantage [PL 94-142, 121a. 5(9)].

Diagnostically, learning disabled children may have a severe discrepancy between achievement and intellectual ability in any or several of these areas:

1. Oral expression
2. Listening comprehension
3. Written expression
4. Basic reading skills
5. Reading comprehension
6. Mathematics calculation
7. Mathematics reasoning

These areas of discrepancy are often revealed by identifying the students' capacity to learn, their achievement, their medical and emotional status, and the internal processing problems. Because there are many learning disabilities a student may exhibit, the authors have decided to concentrate solely on a discussion of the child with severe reading problems. Other learning disabilities involving areas such as writing, spelling, or performing mathematical calculations will be left for future discussion by other professionals.

The law requires that the determination of specific learning disability as a handicap must be made by a multidisciplinary team. At least one member of the team must be a person who is qualified to conduct individual diagnostic examinations of children, including the assessment of aptitude and achievement. Present federal regulations stipulate that this team may determine that a child has a specific learning disability if: (1) the child does not achieve commensurate with his or her age and ability level in one or more of the areas of oral expression, listening comprehension, written expression, basic reading skills, reading comprehension, mathematics calculation, and mathematics reasoning; or (2) the team finds that a child has a severe discrepancy between achievement and intellectual ability in one or more of the above areas.

It is to be recognized that some children whose aptitude is below average will be slow in many skill areas. These children may be learning disabled although their learning characteristics may not conform to existing federal definitions.

In evaluating school children with a learning dysfunction the search for a specific etiology has rarely been successful. In this sense a strict medical model approach is not useful and is not recommended in this book. However, certain medical procedures, such as obtaining a birth history, can prove helpful in identifying "risk factors." For example, infants born prematurely with a low birth weight or with a history of exposure to drugs, trauma, and prolonged labor, have a higher incidence of learning disabilities.

Traditionally and still today, diagnostic procedures frequently result in individual disciplines tending to "guard their own turf" while viewing their own discipline as being central. Ideally, however, the medical team should assist the educator in identifying physical, neurological, and emotional factors that may predispose the child to failure; parents should expect an evaluation that is free from bias, which may be inherent in some school evaluations; and professional clinicians should be called upon when needed. The assessment should include a detailed early history including the pregnancy and perinatal period, early developmental motor and language milestones, family information, and psychological testing. It should also include a clear account of present educational progress, behavioral parameters, and past current emotional status. Additional information can be extrapolated from standardized rating systems, a description of school and home settings, and a complete physical examination.

The diagnosis should be able to describe a child on six levels:

1. Neurodevelopmental: with an evaluation of constitutional and maturational factors
2. Psychosocial: with an emphasis on factors in the family, environment, and past experiences of the child
3. Psychologic: with an insight into effects of failure on the ego
4. Supportive: with a view as to how the family and school cope with the child's disability

5. Coping: with strategies or an analysis of the way the child deals with failure
6. Educational: with an academic profile of a student's strengths and weaknesses.

Medical personnel should be supportive of the educator and should be generally aware of some educational strategies. More importantly, they should know whom to consult for further information. By being knowledgeable, they can more fully and accurately participate in the program planning of the disabled student.

In summary, the role of medicine in reading disability is essentially the same as in any systemic disease. While many severely disabled readers are first referred to a physician, and more specifically an opthalmologist, only infrequently is it primarily a medical or ocular problem. The solution of the problem requires coordinated efforts of many disciplines. The physician, neurologist, psychiatrist, otologist, and ophthalmologist, together with the educator, hearing and speech specialist, occupational and physical therapist, and psychologist, all play important and correlated roles in investigation, solution, and management. Remediation in the final analysis should center about the educator, but a worthy assist is to be had from the other disciplines mentioned above.

There are a multitude of reasons why children do not acquire reading and other language skills despite the fact that no known physical disability is apparent and average or above average cognitive potential exists. This book attempts to explore those multiple factors related to a child's failure in reading through examination of educational, medical, and theoretical viewpoints.

Because there is and will continue to be much confusion and debate among professionals who work with children with reading problems, input from interdisciplinary practitioners in the field is mandatory and has been actively sought in the development of this book. Contemporary and historical references are provided at the end of each chapter so the reader can continue to explore ideas or concerns of his or her interest. Finally, definitions are provided at the end of this book for those who wish to understand those technical terms that are presented in specific chapters.

REFERENCES

Goldberg, H., and Schiffman, G. *Dyslexia: Problems of Reading Disabilities*. New York: Grune & Stratton, 1972

2

Early Predictive Studies

The ability to read is probably more important today than it has been at any other time in history. For centuries, reading was not essential to an agrarian livelihood; thus that ability was primarily used to enhance social and economic status. With the invention of the printing press, urbanization, and industrialization, the ability to read gradually became imperative to greater numbers of people. As the modern world developed, its scientific discoveries and communicative innovations, its intellectual controversies and expanding literary output, and its demand for popular education produced strong pressures for more people to read more printed material.

Certainly, the 1980s will be viewed as part of the most rapidly changing era in history. As science and modern technology continue to influence us, our lives become forced into more and more complicated patterns and the research for knowledge continues to escalate.

Most of us like to read for relaxation and enjoyment and for the satisfaction of being well read. "Keeping up" demands that the individual accumulate more knowledge through the interpretation of written material than has ever been necessary before. A truly vast amount of reading is now required just to maintain proficiency in one's work and to try to solve the perplexing problems of modern society.

As one reviews historical milestones in reading, the complexity

5

of the reading process becomes obvious. In 1877, Kussmaul called attention to a phenomenon that he called "word blindness," and which refers to an individual who is unable to read, although vision, intellect, and speech are unimpaired. In 1896, Morgan published the case of a young boy of average intelligence who had great difficulty in learning the letters of the alphabet; only with the greatest effort could he spell out monosyllabic words, and the configuration of the words appeared to convey little meaning to him. Additionally, there was no impairment of his mathematic abilities. Morgan's report was the first which was not associated with à history of neurologic problems.

There have been other reports of similar cases. Gradually, the condition, originally called *alexia,* was termed *dyslexia,* and today it is often referred to as a specific learning disability. The heterogeneity of students who manifest specific learning disabilities has made identification and remediation complex.

Orton (1937) designated dyslexic children as being delayed in reading compared to achievement in other subjects, whose attempts at reading were characterized by frequent reversals and by confusion between commonly used words such as "saw" and "was," and who showed a greater facility for mirror reading than normal readers. The frequency of reversals caused Orton to suggest the word *strephosymbolia,* meaning "twisted symbols."

In this era of emphasis upon universal and lifelong education, the critical importance of the ability to read well, and with comprehension, becomes clearer when we realize that during the later school years almost 90 percent of a student's studies depend directly upon reading ability. Students who fail to develop highly skilled reading abilities are faced with a serious handicap in their future as productive citizens. The more obvious disadvantages of being a poor reader often include lower lifetime earnings, less social status, and fewer of the possessions and ideals commonly associated with happiness and success in our culture.

Unfortunately, reading problems have also been associated with many serious consequences. For example, poor reading and juvenile delinquency appear to be positively correlated, and children who are considered to be "problem children" are often below average in reading ability. Many educators have concluded that nonreading may very well be an early symptom of antagonism and aggression against discipline and authority. The frustrated nonreader rebels and falls further behind in reading, becoming even more disturbed and antisocial. This growing inadequacy makes it difficult for participation in regular classroom activities, thus increasing alienation from peer groups, which may lead to continued failure and misconduct.

While the terms learning disabilities or dyslexia tend to be ambiguous, "reading" itself is a term of even greater ambiguity. It is little wonder that research studies in reading are subject to contradictory interpretation.

Early studies of dyslexia were confusing due to the wide variation of definitions. Historically, terms often used synonymously with dyslexia included: *primary reading disability, specific developmental dyslexia, congenital word blindness, strephosymbolia, specific reading disability,* and *developmental lag.*

Today, a general agreement exists that there is no single etiology for a child with specific learning disabilities. The majority of these children do, however, have average or above average intelligence, an absence of sensory deficits, an absence of gross neurological impairment, and often have had conventional teaching thought to be adequate for the development of reading. Some authors do not specify that average or above average intelligence is a necessary requisite, since many children might still have a language disability superimposed on an inadequate capacity to learn.

The estimates of reading failure may include up to 10 to 20 percent of the school population. This percentage applies to the average school system with perhaps a higher incidence of failure in inner city or rural school systems. While some professionals might disagree, there is no single technique which remediates the problem of specific learning disability.

Many excellent books have been written on a variety of reading difficulties (Adamson and Adamson, 1979; Johnson and Myklebust, 1967; Bond and Tinker, 1967). The majority of this material, however, addresses the educational process with teaching methods and remediation suggestions. With all that has been written, there is still very little authoritative data available on the basic causes of reading disability. This is true to a great extent because the process of reading is extremely complex, and, therefore, not fully understood.

Reading with understanding is a complicated procedure involving educational, psychological, physiological, and anatomical factors. Both the learning process and those conditions that may inhibit it will be discussed in greater detail in later chapters.

The failure of some children to progress in reading with an ability commensurate with others of their own age has been the subject of a great amount of controversy. Because so little is known about this area, a child's inability to interpret written material successfully has been attributed to a number of factors. Vision (see Chapter 6) has been cited as a cause of this problem, with many individuals indicating that it is due to the eye muscles not functioning properly. Others assail heredity (see Chapter 10) as the cause. Some say that poor reading is related to lack of cerebral dominance (see Chapter 4). Still other observers blame diseases of the blood. Even the improper functioning of the thyroid gland and of other ductless glands have been mentioned as causes of reading deficiency. The fact remains that none of these assumptions has been adequately substantiated.

Basic to a comprehension of reading problems is an understanding of the term "reading readiness." Each child who begins school has a varied and different physical, emotional, and educational profile. Traditionally, at the moment children reach 5 or 6 years of age, the parents, teacher, and society expect them to be ready for reading.

Under ideal conditions, children are prepared to make an easy transition from oral language to written language. They learn to listen, then to talk; they learn to organize language in the form of sentences and paragraphs. This combination of concepts, attitudes, and interests provides the foundation upon which reading ability is built, and with each child there is some variation in the facility he or she shows for reading readiness. At the "strategic" age of 5 or 6 years, many factors might influence or delay the coordinated development of reading skill and play a prominent part in the causation of a reading problem.

In many instances, children with specific learning disabilities have been considered lazy and unwilling to learn. Parents and teachers may have recognized that they are intelligent, especially in areas that interest them. They may do well in out-of-school activities that require an alert, intelligent mind, thus causing parents and teachers to reach the erroneous conclusion that they are not trying to do well in school. They become convinced that a bit of determined effort is all that is required. Children of this type have traditionally not been promoted in school, possibly as punishment for their "laziness," but possibly in an honest effort to shock them into putting forth an effort to learn. In addition, their parents (see Chapter 5) may have restricted their outside activities in order to have them do extra school work and may have drilled them on work assigned for the next day. The main result is nearly always a totally frustrated parent and child.

Furthermore, special reading instruction has often been subject to the advocacy of faddists who offer many types of remediation suggestions, with little thought given to the primary causes of the reading disturbance. It is not only teachers, but reading clinicians, other professionals, and parents who often use terms such as "emotional block," "minimal brain damage (MBD)," and "brain damage" to dismiss a problem that they do not understand.

The number of children with learning disabilities is increasing, and as the number increases so does the complexity of the problem. Denhoff and Hainsworth (1972) has found that 10 percent of children in middle-class homes risk school failure in the first three grades. This figure is stated to be 20 to 40 percent in some local school systems.

Predictive studies (Rubin and Balow, 1980, and Francis-Williams, 1976) should assist in providing an answer as to why some children progress slowly in the learning situation and why some children consistently have difficulty and are never able to return to the regular mainstream of education. We now know that identical methods of teaching should not be applied to all children, since the causes of learning disabilities are very heterogeneous and a "paint spray" approach will only lead to confusion.

The greatest strength of early predictive diagnosis is that it may result in a preventive approach which avoids or minimizes learning disabilities before failure is entrenched.

Ideally, children with real or potential learning difficulties should be identified before beginning school or certainly by first grade. If this could be accomplished, teachers would be able to outline for the children an academic program that could be adjusted to the maximum ways in which they could learn and perhaps at a pace at which learning should proceed. The growing number of children with reading disabilities make it imperative that there should be some way to assess their cognitive capacities so adjustments could be made to coincide more realistically with their aptitudes. Therefore, one of our most important contributions in dealing with the problem of reading disabilities may well be in the area of early predictive studies.

Psychologists and educators have always sought a measure which would sort out and differentiate the capabilities of school students. Millions of children take intelligence tests every year. Some critics say that these tests are culturally biased and that the component tests do not add up to a measure of intelligence.

The first tests of mental measurement were designed by Sir Francis Galton (1889), who attempted to prove that intelligence was inherited. In 1905 the French psychologist, Alfred Binet, developed a series of tests to identify mentally defective children. Following the administration of his tests to large numbers of children of various ages, he derived the concept of "mental age." Lewis M. Terman, an American psychologist, later developed the concept of "intelligence quotient." By dividing the mental age of the child by his chronological age and multiplying the result by 100, one could obtain the IQ (intelligence quotient) scores of the child. Terman revised the Binet test so as to identify the most capable children in order that they could have educational and cultural advantages that would prepare them for leadership. This revision was known as the Stanford-Binet Test (Terman and Merrill, 1961).

It must be remembered that an intelligence test is meaningful only under carefully controlled conditions of individual testing by a certified psychologist, who can bring out the best of a child's ability to perform and who can remain sensitive to the level of the child's motivation during the testing situation.

An IQ score, furthermore, is not a fixed score. Fluctuations can occur because of physical, emotional, and cultural changes. Most recently, it has been found that children from homes that provided poor cognitive stimulation do poorly on intelligence tests.

Stress during the first year of life has been found to be related to learning disabilities (Denhoff and Hainsworth, 1972). Evaluation of stress includes complications during pregnancy, elevated blood pressure, proteinuria, convulsions, trauma, intoxications, socio-environmental conditions, respiratory distress, dysmaturity, low-birth weight, high-bilirubin level, and haemolytic syndromes. Children who are evaluated at 7 years of age and who are frequently unsuccessful in school tend to have had higher scores on stress indices.

When investigating children in a John Hopkins collaborative project Hardy (1971) found high APGAR scores, elevated bilirubin blood levels, and a birth weight below 1500 grams. These were all correlated to minimal brain dysfunction, lower intelligence, and reading failure.

Historically, in 1935 Castner attempted to identify reasons related to reading failure in the young child. In 1966 DeHirsch published a book on early predictive studies in which she attempted to identify children who might have difficulties in the school system. Her purpose was not only to predict success or failure but to offer suggestions on how to help the child who might be a high-risk student in the normal learning situation. It was suggested that this high-risk child could become a successful reader and experience success devoid of frustration.

A pilot study of the feasibility of early prediction by DeHirsch, Jansky and Langford (1966) sought to determine which of 50 or so children at the kindergarten level were likely to fail in reading two years later. First, they presented 37 variables to these kindergarten children. The product of these 37 tests was a 10-test battery called the Predictive Index. This index was the result of those tests given in kindergarten that had the highest coefficient of correlation with second-grade reading, as well as those that best separated the failing readers from the remainder of the group. The 10 tests found to make up the Predictive Index were (1) Pencil Use, (2) Bender Motor Gestalt, (3) Wepman Auditory Discrimination, (4) Categories, (5) Number of Words Used in Telling a Story, (6) the Word Matching subtest of the Gates Reading Readiness Battery, (7) the Horst Matching Test, (8) two Word Learning tests, (9) a Spelling Learning task, and (10) Letter Naming tests.

Of the original group of kindergarten children, these 10 tests had identified 10 of the 11 children who subsequently failed reading at the end of the second grade. Upon completion of this study, it was evident that an effort would have to be made to validate these tests, that is, to give the tests to a much larger sampling of children in order to determine their general usefulness and reliability as early predictors. This research was carried out by Jansky (1971) who undertook the second phase of early prediction research.

By the time the research plan for the second study was being formulated, a number of people had already started to use the Predictive Index. It was desirable to devise such a battery because professionals were seeking a shorter instrument, which could easily be administered by school personnel; also, there was much interest in trying several measures not included among the 37 kindergarten tests originally administered to children in the first study. Thus, while it was planned to validate the Predictive Index on a second group of children, the major concern of phase 2 shifted to the preparation of a shorter instrument that would conceivably be useful to more people.

The subjects for the second study were kindergarten children drawn from 5 public schools in 2 districts of New York City. The kindergarten tests were administered to all children who spoke and understood conversational English. Of the group of 508 children tested as kindergarteners, 341 continued to attend the schools in which they had originally been enrolled and were available for evaluation 2 years later. Sixty more of the original group were located, so that the final sample consisted of 401 subjects to whom both kindergarten and second grade tests had been administered.

About 50 percent of the children were white, 42 percent were black, while the remaining were Puerto Rican or Chinese.

The kindergarten tests were administered individually to the children at their schools in the spring of the kindergarten year. Additional tests were included to increase the number of measures in certain categories. These were Letter Naming Test, Number of Words Used in Telling a Story, the Minnesota Perceptual Diagnostic Test (which involved the copying of designs and calculating the extent to which they were rotated), Sentence Memory Items (from the 1937 Stanford-Binet), a Picture Naming task, the Roswell-Chall Auditory Blending Test, a clinical assessment of Oral Language Level, and a measure of the child's tendency to use Configuration for Word Matching.

The first problem of the second phase of this research was to see how the Predictive Index would apply with a new group of children. Some conclusions drawn from the findings in the second testing and relating to validation of the Predictive Index developed in the first study may be summarized as follows. The old Predictive Index varied in efficiency when used with new samples. The accuracy with which the failing readers were identified varied from sample to sample. Because of population differences, norms changed within the individual school and norms developed for one population did not hold for another. The Predictive Index as used with the heterogeneous group of 300 kindergarten children was most efficient in preselecting the best of the second grade readers. The Predictive Index also seemed to function most efficiently in identifying the failing readers when used with children whose IQ clustered around 100. When administered to the subgroup of 50 children matched to first-study subjects, the Index's performance was satisfactory and the results were nearly identical to those of the earlier research.

The major goal of the second study was to devise a screening test that could be administered quickly and that would, therefore, be useful for large, heterogeneous populations. As with the first study, a cutoff point was selected that resulted in identifying as many actual reading failures and in introducing as few false positives (children who later passed) as possible.

In Jansky's second efforts, a group of five tests was selected as predictors. The battery developed included the Letter Naming, Picture Naming tests, the Gates Word Matching, the Bender Motor Gestalt, and the Sentence Memory tests as additional contributors. This short screening battery correctly identified 79 percent of the failing readers. It identified only 22 percent of the children who actually passed.

To achieve high accuracy rates in individual prediction it is essential to take advantage of the kindergarten teachers' knowledge of the children. In the process of formulating clinical predictions, the teachers weigh all they know about a child to arrive at their prognostication of the child's future development. Although teachers' predictions alone are not sufficient, they do represent a valuable source of information to be checked against so-called "hard" data. There is no need to view clinical and statistical prediction as mutually exclusive.

"SOFT SIGNS" AS PREDICTORS

Soft signs refer to those deficits in age-appropriate performance of certain neurologically mediated tasks that are not usually identified in the traditional neurological examination.

The relevance of soft signs (Adams et. al., 1974, Hart et. al., 1974) in identifying children with learning disabilities remains controversial. The evaluation of these signs may be relevant in identifying groups of neurologically handicapped children, as evidenced by the differentiation of normal and language-impaired children, but it is unclear whether the presence of such soft signs in an individual child can, of themselves, be a significant contributor to the planning of intervention strategies or the predicting of outcomes.

The normal function of the cerebral cortex is dependent on the integrity of connections (synapses) between neurons. The interneuronal connections have been called "neuronal circuitry." Because there is insufficient pathological material we must examine neuronal circuitry in animals.

One of the most difficult diagnostic problems facing the communication disorders specialist is that of assessing the potential for language development in the child who is not yet speaking. Among the prespeech language-related skills that need to be assessed in this context are auditory processing and speech perception skills.

Studies (Stark and Tallal, 1981) of auditory processing abilities in normal and language-delayed children have indicated that: (1) these perception abilities are significantly depressed in children with language disorders as compared with normal children; (2) speech perception abilities are highly correlated with measures of receptive language in school-age language-disordered children; and (3) speech perception abilities are not innate but appear to develop with age in both normal and language-delayed children. These findings suggest that it is very important to develop measures of speech perception abilities that could be employed in the assessment of individual children in the first two years of life. Such measures would make it possible to determine whether or not, in infants and very young children, delays in development of speech perception are predictive of later language disorders.

Unfortunately the measures of speech perception in infants that have been developed to date indicate that speech perception abilities are not innate but must be developed. At present, an indication of auditory processing impairments in otherwise normal infants and young children may be derived from simple tests of comprehension of language. Such measures may make it possible to identify children who are of normal intelligence, but yet at risk for language disorders, from a very early age, even before they would be expected to talk in single words or phrases. Early identification, in turn, would make it possible to initiate language intervention at an early age and ultimately to assess the effectiveness of such early intervention.

Ertl and Barry (1966) in a controversial approach, used the visually evoked response (VER) as a possible method of gaining learning disability information. The VER was done by exposing the child to tachistoscopic stimuli while electrodes recorded the electrical sensations received in the brain. These individual responses were computerized, summated, and averaged, and the final VER wave produced. Connors (1970–1971) described a family of poor readers who had a change in the wave form of the visually evoked response in the left parietal area of the brain. Studies of two samples of poor readers, and a sample of children with contrasting verbal-performance discrepancies on the Wechsler Intelligence Scale for Children (WISC, original version) showed significant relationships between verbal skills and the late components of the VER. The strongest VER amplitude correlations appear to have occurred in the left parietal area. Children with verbal-performance discrepancies on the WISC also showed highly significant latency effects in the late waves of the VER.

Amplitude changes of wave forms in the left parietal area suggest an alteration in the information processing capabilities of this area in reading disorders. Test data indicate that children with low performance IQs are more impaired neurologically and thus would have poorer results on the performance part of the WISC. Although it is too early to be certain, the VER might be an instrument that could be used in early identification of children with learning disability. Subsequent investigations should provide more information as to the reliability of the VER and its role in the investigation of learning disabilities.

In summary, there is a clear need for accurate prediction. Considering what we already know about children and the objective measures of their relative performance on tests, it may be possible to conclude that tests are available that may have predictive ability as they relate to reading success. It must be remembered, however, that prediction involves interpreting relevant information about the child and considering it systematically, and this information can only be accurate to the degree that it is highly individualized.

The purpose of predictive tests at the preschool or primary level should include differentiating children of varying learning capacities, as well as identifying specific areas of handicapping conditions. The prospects of remedial success are greatly improved if the children's learning disabilities can be recognized before they become enmeshed in a pattern of frustration and failure. One of the purposes of this book is to encourage the identification of the contributing factors in a learning disability, such as visual, auditory, neurological, or educational factors. Equally important is the attempt to present persuasive evidence for the need to understand a child's strengths and deficiencies so that teaching efforts may be enhanced and probabilities increased for attaining educational goals.

REFERENCES

Adams, R., Kocsis, J., and Estes, R. Soft neurological signs in learning disabled children and controls. *American Journal of Disabled Children,* 1974, *128,* 614−618.

Adamson, W., and Adamson, K. *A handbook for specific learning disabilities.* New York: Gardner Press, Inc. 1979.

Apgar, V., and Beck, J. *Is my baby all right?* New York: Trident Press, 1972.

Binet, A. *L'ame et le corps.* Paris: E. Flammarion, 1905.

Bond, G. and Tinker, M. *Reading difficulties: Their diagnosis and correction.* Englewood Cliffs, N.J. Prentice-Hall, 1967.

Castner, B. Prediction of reading disability prior to first grade entrance. *American Journal of Orthopsychiatry,* 1935, *5:* 375−387.

Connors, C. Cortically visual-evoked responses in children with learning disabilities. *Psychophysiology,* 1970−1971, *7,* 418.

DeHirsch, K. Tests designed to discover potential reading difficulties at six year old level. *American Journal of Orthopsychiatry,* 1957, *27,* 566−576.

DeHirsch, K., Jansky, J., and Langford, W. *Predicting reading failure.* New York: Harper and Row, 1966.

Denhoff, E., and Hainsworth, P. The child at risk for learning disorder: Can he be identified during the first years of life? *Clinical Pediatrics.* 1972, *11,* 164−170.

Ertl, J. and Barry, W. Researchers: Quid mine IQ? *M.D. Magazine,* June, 1966.

Flax, N. Visual function in learning disabilities. *Journal of Learning Disabilities,* 1968, *1,* 74−78.

Francis-Williams, J. Early identification of children likely to have specific learning difficulties. *Developmental Medicine and Child Neurology,* 1976, *18,* 71−77.

Galton, F. *Natural inheritance.* London: Macmillan & Company, 1889.

Hardy, J., and Peeples, M. Serum bilirubin levels in newborn infants: Distributions and associations with neurological abnormalities during the first year of life. *John Hopkins Medical Journal,* 1971, *128,* 265−272.

Hart, Z., Rennick, P., Klinge, V., and Schwartz, M. A pediatric neurologist's contributions to evaluations of school underachievers. *American Journal of Disabled Children.* 1974, *128*, 319–323.

Johnson D., and Myklebust, H. *Learning disabilities: Educational principles and practices.* New York: Grune & Stratton, Inc., 1976.

Kussmaul, A. Disturbance of speech. *Cyclopedia of Practical Medicine,* 1977, *14*, 581–875.

Mark, H. *Brain damage in children etiology-diagnosis-treatment.* Baltimore, Maryland: Williams and Wilkens Publishing Company.

Morgan, W. A case of congenital word blindness. *British Medical Journal,* 1896, *2*, 1378–1379.

Orton, S. *Reading, writing and speech problems in children.* New York: W. W. Norton & Company, 1937.

Palmer, F., Capute, A., Shapiro, B., and Accardo, P. Linguistic development between 12–24 months: A cognitive predictor. *Pediatric Research,* in press.

Rawson, M. Bibliography on the nature, recognition and treatment of language difficulties. *Bulletin of the Orton Society,* 1971.

Rubin, R., and Balow, B. Infant neurological abnormalities as indicators of cognitive impairment. *Developmental Medicine and Child Neurology,* 1980, *22*, 336–343.

Schiffman, G., and Clemmons, R. *Observations on children with severe reading problems and learning disorders.* Seattle, Washington: Special Child Publications, 1966.

Seiderman, A. Under scruting of optometry. *Pediatrics,* 1976, *57*, 980–981.

Slingerland, B. *Screening test for identifying children with specific learning disabilities.* Cambridge, Mass: Educators Publishing Service, 1969.

Solan, H. Physiological correlates of dyslexia. *American Journal of Optometry and Archives of American Academy of Optometry,* 1966, *43*, 3–9.

Stark, R., and Tallal, P. Perceptual and motor deficits in language impaired children. In R. W. Keith (Ed.), *Central auditory and language disorders in children.* Houston: College Hill Press, 1981.

Terman, E., and Merrill, M. *Stanford-Binet intelligence scale, manual for third revision.* Boston: Houghton-Mifflin Co., 1961.

3

Psychological Evaluation

The reading disabled child is one who demonstrates an inability to read at expectancy using the child's intellectual endowment as the bench mark for the level of expectancy. It is also assumed that the discrepancy between a child's ability to read and the expectancy is caused by an underlying psychoneurological difficulty or dysfunction, which interferes significantly with the processes necessary for reading to be functionally adequate.

Severe reading disability or dyslexia is not a simple syndrome with one etiology; it is a dysfunction or delay, and the underlying basis of the disorder is the brain, not a poor environment, poor parenting, poor teaching, difficulties in gross motor balance, or difficulties in visual tracking. Personality problems or emotional disorders may compound the disability, but children who are poor readers because they are emotionally disturbed are not dyslexic. Any of these problems can exist in combination, and good diagnostic evaluations are necessary to best factor out the causes since the causes frequently determine the focus of treatment and remediation.

The multi-factor hypotheses of Birch (1962) and Myklebust (1962) state that the constitutional disorder causing *dyslexic* reading difficulties results in symptoms that are significantly different in many qualitative ways from other reading problems. The underlying psychological processes involving auditory and visual perception, memory, and sequencing seem to be at the core of these qualitative differences noted in Chapters 6 and 8. The psychological evaluation attempts to sample these and other psychological processes. The neurochemical, neuroanatomical dysfunctions or deficits that may produce these process problems are not as yet clearly identified. There is no known way of predicting severe reading disability in children or infants even if they have known pre- or post-natal minimal neurological trauma. Children can be targeted as "at risk" of having this specific learning disability prior to entering school. However, aside from stimulation programs that are frequently geared to children from homes where pre-academic infant stimulation is not the norm, there is little evidence that much improves the reading ability of these minimally "at risk" children. Certainly children who are late talkers and who have language disabilities prior to entering school are at greater risk of being reading disabled than children whose language development has been normal (Stark, 1981). When talking about language disabled children, we are assuming that language is severely deficient, again using intelligence as the bench mark. The work of Jansky and DeHirsch (1972) has shown some promise in predicting difficulty in reading among preschool age children with language deficits.

Measurements of cognitive ability are most accurately determined by psychometric evaluations carried out by qualified psychologists whose specialty involves these types of assessment. Psychologists qualified to carry out psychometric testing are generally clinical psychologists, school psychologists, educational psychologists, and counseling psychologists who are certified and/or licensed and who generally work in clinics or public schools or in private practice or in other private facilities. Psychological evaluations always go beyond the mere assessment of cognitive functioning and most frequently include assessments of personality factors and perceptual motor functioning, as well as motivation and attention. The psychologist does not utilize the psychometric techniques merely as standardized measures of the child's intellectual, perceptual, motoric, and emotional well being, but has the ethical responsibility to view these samples of behavior in the light of the child's developmental history and physiological integrity, as well as family, home, and school environmental influences. Determination must be made as to the appropriateness of techniques to be utilized and as to the tests that measure the components of the assessment in relation to their appropriateness for the individual child. It is known that test bias can result in significant errors in the predictive usefulness of data. Jane Mercer (1979) has demonstrated that IQ tests are culturally biased toward white middle-class males and show a significant negative bias toward minority groups, such as Spanish Americans, blacks, and American Indians, as well as any socioculturally "different" persons. According to her studies sociocultural factors accounted for as much as "32 percent of the variance in IQ scores in a sample of 1,513 elementary school children." In everyday language this means that if you knew the child's sociocultural level, then you would have a better chance of accurately predicting the IQ results than if you knew another general fact about the child. Mercer does not deny the importance of assessment in determining if the organism is intact (medical component), but she separates this diagnostic question from the behavioral-social component of the individual and the prediction of the individual's learning potential (intelligence). Mercer objects to the collapse of these distinct reasons for assessment. Many of Mercer's points are important, but there remains a significant amount of research that suggests that careful analysis of the IQ test data used in conjunction with other assessment material can provide significant medically collaborative information. Furthermore, regardless of sociocultural-economic background, neurological factors do affect functioning on IQ tests such as the Wechsler Intelligence Scale for Children-Revised (WISC-R). Many researchers have shown strong relationships between neurological dysfunctions, special education problems, and the results on the WISC-R.

COMMONLY USED PSYCHOLOGICAL
EVALUATION MEASURES

The purpose of the psychological evaluation is to provide information that will improve on the probability of making the best decision for treatment, program, or educational planning. The psychological evaluation is only one component in the diagnostic and prescriptive process. Great errors have been made by practitioners and researchers alike using psychometric results as "the" criterion for prescription or prediction.

There is a general battery of techniques used by psychologists in this evaluation process, which include observation, interview, history gathering, and psychometric measures. Most teachers and other professionals focus on the psychometric measures when they think of the psychological evaluation, since many of these instruments are viewed as the most valid parts of the battery. However, it is frequently the subjective information secured through history, interview, record review, and observation that guides the psychologist in judging the validity of the psychometric samples of behavior.

The psychometric measure most frequently used for the evaluation of intelligence of school-age children is the Wechsler Intelligence Scale for Children-Revised (WISC-R), (Wechsler, 1974). A survey reported at the 1980 National Association of School Psychologists Convention indicated that the WISC-R is used nearly 80 percent of the time for the assessment of intelligence in school-age children (Goh, Teslow, & Fuller, 1980). Other frequently used intelligence measures, such as the Stanford Binet (third revision), are more commonly applied to questions of retardation than of dyslexia or learning problems. The WISC-R is standardized for the age range of 6 years 0 months through 16 years 11 months. As with any test, when approaching the lower or upper age limits, it may be useful to use another instrument for validating purposes. Many psychologists report that the WICS-R is less useful as a test for younger children in providing a rich sample of behavior. Wechsler (1967) developed the Wechsler Preschool and Primary Scale of Intelligence (WPPSI) to meet this concern. The WPPSI provides a comparable measure for youngsters age 4 years through 6 years 6 months. Both the WPPSI and WISC-R provide Verbal and Performance Scale IQs, a point that has been highly valued in factoring out the two primary components of what we call "general intelligence." David Wechsler defines general intelligence as "the overall capacity of an individual to understand and cope with the world around him" (Wechsler, 1974 [Manual, p. 5]).

The concept of general intelligence is demonstrated on these tests in that all of their subtests show positive relationships with each other. There are many other intelligence tests used in assessing children and some of these have great merit, including the Columbia Mental Maturity Scale (1972). There are measures, such as the Peabody Picture Vocabulary Test (1959), which may measure receptive vocabulary but does not measure what we call general intelligence. Other tests, such as the Slosson Intelligence Test (Slosson, 1971), may measure more aspects of general intelligence but seem to lack the refined statistical standardization desired by psychologists.

Standardization means more than just administering the test in a standard way, each time providing time limits and no cues beyond the instructions. Standardization means that the test is normed on a clearly representative sample of the population for each age group for which the test is standardized. Representation must take into consideration all factors that are known about the population that could influence results, including sex, race, geographic region, urban and rural residence, and occupation of head of the household. In the case of the WISC-R, for example, each age group sample (ages 6 ½ through 16 ½) contains a representative number of individuals using the 1970 U.S. Census as the reference group for the above variables. This is called a stratified sample and is similar to those used in political polls. There are some vital factors not dealt with in any standardization that could significantly influence results, including many orthopaedic problems as well as deafness and blindness. Using the test norms for these and other children for whom the test was not standardized is unethical. Many other intervening variables can influence test results, such as the child's inability to understand the nature of the task, test anxiety, lack of familiarity with the significance of the test, or even temporary illness unknown to the examiner. These variables are believed to be evenly distributed and therefore controlled by the size and representativeness of the standardization sample. For the WISC-R, normalizing the results means counting the number of correct responses on each subtest at each age level and converting this raw score to a scale in which the average number of correct responses for their age is given a score of 10 and a standard deviation of 3. Sixty-seven percent of the children in that age group have raw scores that fall within the scale score range of 7 through 13. WISC-R IQ's are based upon these subtest scale scores. Verbal, Performance, and Full Scale IQs from 85 through 115 would account for the same 67 percent. The IQ of 100 is defined as the performance of the average child at any specific age. Intelligence is classified as follows in Table 3-1 (Weschler, 1974 [Manual, p. 26]):

Along with standardization, a test can only be viewed as a useful predictor if it is reliable, has a small error of measurement and is valid in measuring what it purports to measure and predict. The

Table 3-1
WISC-R Intelligence Classifications

I.Q. Score	Classification	Percent of Normal Curve
130+	Very Superior	2.2
120–129	Superior	6.7
110–119	High Average	16.1
90–109	Average	50.0
80–89	Low Average	16.1
70–79	Borderline	6.7
69 and below	Mentally Deficient	2.2

WISC-R meets these requirements. As Nadine Lambert (1981) states, "Recent extensive reviews of all available tests used for special education purposes have shown that the WISC-R is probably the most valid, fairest, and surely the most studied of any instrument in the school psychologist's list." Using the WISC-R as a valid predictor of dyslexia involves taking a close look at the pattern of subtest scores. The previously long-standing comparison of Verbal and Performance IQ's in determining the existence of this learning problem has been discarded as too simplistic. Present practitioners follow an analysis of the 12 subtests, grouping them according to intellectual processes. Bannatyne (1974) is probably the best-known reorganizer of the Wechsler scales.

A review of the WISC-R subtests may help familiarize the reader with this revised breakdown. The Verbal subtests include:

1. *Information* (30 items). This subtest is composed of a wide spectrum of basic fact questions that measure the individual's ability to recall facts that have been acquired from experience and education. It correlates highly with academic achievement, is significantly affected by experiential background, memory difficulties, auditory problems, emotional and attitudinal problems, as well as general mental deficiency.

2. *Similarities* (17 items). This subtest is composed of pairs of words that require recognition of likenesses ranging from the concrete to the abstract. It measures conceptual ability and associative thinking. General mental deficiency affects this subtest as well as problems in shifting one's thinking and forming inferences.

3. *Arithmetic* (18 items). This subtest requires mental computation in response to word problems. It requires focusing attention on the sequence of the information in the question, short-term memory and reorganization (translation) of verbal material into numerical operations. There is a time limit. The results are affected by anxiety as well as difficulties in maintaining focused attention and shifting thinking. Sequencing problems depress scores on this subtest. Poor experience may also be a factor.
4. *Vocabulary* (32 words, primarily nouns). This subtest requires definitions and again moves from the concrete identification level to the abstract. Of all the subtests, vocabulary correlates best with general intelligence and is also a good predictor of academic achievement. It measures verbal conceptualization and is affected by language skills as well as experience.
5. *Comprehension* (17 items). The responses to the questions in this subtest hinge on judgment in combination with practical knowledge of social situations. It measures conceptual thinking and coping skills sometimes called commonsense reasoning. Many of the questions are relatively complex, and therefore receptive language skills are needed to correctly "hear" the questions. Serious emotional problems and poor reality testing, as well as limited experience, depress scores on this subtest as does general mental deficiency. Some impulsive responders have difficulty with this subtest due to auditory attention problems.
6. *Digit Span* (14 number series). This is a supplemental subtest that is crucial to proper subtest analysis but is not included in obtaining the IQs. A series of numbers given at 1 per second must be repeated in order. It also requires repeating a series of numbers backwards. This subtest measures sequential short-term memory (recall). It requires attention and freedom from distractibility. It is affected by anxiety as well as specific processing problems in aural sequencing. It is less affected by experience and does not correlate well with general intelligence. It may be the highest scale score for some youngsters who are mentally deficient.

The Performance Scale is also divided into 6 subtests, of which one, the Mazes, is a supplement. The subtests are:

1. *Picture Completion* (26 incomplete pictures). This subtest requires the child to identify verbally or by pointing out the

important missing element of the picture. It measures visual discrimination, visual memory, and ability to focus on the essential. Figure–ground skills and attention to spatial details seem important. Again, impulsive responders have problems with this task as do those with poor reality testing. The perfectionist may do significantly better on this subtest than on the other subtests on the Performance Scale.

2. *Picture Arrangement* (12 series of comic-striplike pictures). In this subtest, pictures are used to make a story, but they are presented out of order. Time limits and time credits are included elements. Task involves visual comprehension, problem-solving judgment, and sensory integration, as well as attention to visual details. As children get older, the norms become increasingly dependent upon speed of responses, which may have little to do with the cognitive process. Again, youngsters with emotional problems and poor reality testing have problems with this subtest.

3. *Block Design* (11 two-color designs constructed from 4 or 9 blocks). The student is required to construct a design from a picture or model. It involves basic nonverbal intelligence and correlates highly with Performance IQ. It is a good measure of visual motor coordination and integration and is influenced by past experience. Youngsters with neurological damage have difficulty with this subtest. Youngsters with figure-ground confusion problems also have difficulty with this task. Since time limits and time bonuses are elements of this task, youngsters who are lethargic or overly reflective may not do well, particularly among teenagers, when time credits become more crucial.

4. *Object Assembly* (4 puzzles of familiar objects). Requires the child to put 5 to 8 pieces together to construct a familiar object. Again involves time limits and bonus time credits. It involves part–whole perceptual organizational skills. Visual-spatial closure skills, speed, and attention are important. Trial and error and intuitive problem-solving styles can be observed. As with the Block Design, this subtest may be diagnostically useful in cases of organic damage, particularly to the right hemisphere.

5. *Coding* (form depends on age, below 8 years, 45 symbols; above 8 years, 95 items). Requires rapid copying of symbols for numerals in a limited time. It relies on speed of movement, accuracy, shifting in visual-motor integration, visual sequential memory, and discrimination. Scores are depressed when there

is poor visual attention to detail coordinated with motor speed. Youngsters who tend to rotate and reverse or perseverate have trouble witth this task. Correlates highly with specific learning disabiliities and difficulties on pencil-paper perceptual motor coordination tasks. Also affected by anxiety and test attitude. Coding does not correlate with general intelligence as high as most other subtests.

6. *Mazes* (optional supplement composed of 9 typical mazes to be completed without lifting the pencil off the paper). Requires visual, perceptual motor coordination and planning. This is a good subtest to analyze a child's ability to plan before moving. This subtest has been viewed as more "culturally fair" than many others. It is the least frequently administered of the 12 subtests. It is sometimes helpful as an additional measure of the child's learning and problem-solving style and may also be useful for validating pencil–paper small muscle coordination problems as well as responses to frustration.

Bannatyne's pattern analysis of the Wechsler Scales divides the scales into four factors as seen in Table 3-2.

Rugel (1974) demonstrated a characteristic profile for reading-disabled children that showed the average of scaled scores of the Spatial factor to be greater than the average for Verbal Conceptual and the scaled score average of Verbal Conceptual greater than the Sequential Factor. These results conform to the Arithmetic, Coding, Information, Digit Span (ACID) factor for learning disabilities, which is well outlined in Kaufman's writings (1975, 1976, 1979, 1981).

Kaufman adds the Information subtest to the Sequential factor suggesting that the scale score average of these four subtests is characteristically lower for the learning disabled than for factor 2 or

Table 3-2

Factor Name	Subtests
Acquired Knowledge	Information, Vocabulary, Arithmetic
Verbal Conceptualization	Similarities, Vocabulary, Comprehension
Spatial	Picture Completion, Block Design, Object Assembly
Sequential	Arithmetic, Digit Span, Coding

3 (see Table 6-1). He supports the factor pattern analysis approach to the subtest scores but also points out the frequently conflicting research results: "The characteristic LD (learning disabled) profile of low scores on the ACID subtests make much more sense when interpreted from Bannatyne's four category approach than from Wechsler's two-scale system" (Kaufman, 1981). Kaufman noted another recent publication that also supports this concept in spite of other conflicting research results. As indicated earlier, when analysis of normed test data results are applied to diagnosis, the process should be validated by examining these results in light of the child's history, experience, and home and school environment. It is the concept of the Bannatyne categorization that seems useful, provided it is not used as a pure statistical analysis. For example, other studies on youngsters with Superior IQs on the WISC-R showed Verbal Conceptual scale scores to be the highest followed by Spatial and then Sequential scores. These children might also show high scores on Information as well. Some psychologists report that this phenomenon found among learning disabled youngsters who have *Superior* intelligence is also evident among youngsters who have *Average* or better intelligence scores and who are from experientially enriched backgrounds. However, the Sequential scaled scores as a group remain the lowest of the three categories.

Psychologists in general look cautiously at the Full Scale IQ on the WISC-R when there is dramatic scatter, either among subtest scores or between the Verbal and Performance scales. (Subtest scale scores can range from a minimum of 1 to a maximum of 19; 10 is the average for the age group, and 3 is the standard deviation.) Surely one can see the difference between a child who has scaled scores in the 9−10−11 range and a Verbal, Performance, and Full Scale IQ of 100, and the youngster who has scaled scores ranging from 4−16 with a Verbal IQ of 120 and a Performance IQ of 84 and a Full Scale IQ of 102. The second child may well be at high risk of having serious neurological problems and surely needs further study. The former youngster may with greater certainty be seen as *Average*.

The Spatial, Conceptual, Sequential pattern has been found to exist among groups of youngsters who have been classified as emotionally disturbed and juvenile delinquents, and these results have been used to criticize this factor approach. However, Campbell's (1979) study sponsored by Educational Testing Services shows that learning disabilities, and particularly serious reading disabilities, are found to occur in the delinquent population two to

three times more frequently than among the regular school population. It is hypothesized by Campbell that the delinquency is frequently the result of reading problems that create a growing sense of
worthlessness and frustration, which is translated into behavior
problems that frequently begin in school. The same is true for the
emotionally disturbed. As one psychologist indicated, "Learning
disabled (dyslexic) children are labeled language disabled when
preschoolers and learning disabled in elementary school and emotionally disturbed when they reach adolescence. The child's problems don't change, only how we look at them and label them"
(Dwyer, 1981).

There is an equally important approach to the sample of
behavior of the WISC-R that defies the analysis of a computer.
Scores on subtests tell us very little about how the child responded,
and it is the quality of the responses, the errors in particular, that are
important to well-trained psychologists. The 9-year-old child who
responds to a question on naming the months of the year with the
days of the week may have a time sequence problem, while a child
who can only remember 10 of the 12 months presents another
problem. The third child who says "I don't know" gives the
psychologist little to analyze. All three children get zero points on
this hypothetical question. The second child may later recall the
names of the other 2 months. The first child may know the names of
the 12 months, but this information may be stored and retrievable
only in another way.

Another frequently used psychometric measure is the assessment battery in the Bender Visual Motor Gestalt Test (BVMGT),
developed by Lauretta Bender in 1938. This pencil-paper copying
test involves copying nine two-dimensional geometric designs.
Standardized by Koppitz (1964) for children ages 5 through 11, the
test has been viewed as a valid instrument for assisting in screening
neurologically impaired children from normal children, particularly
if specific errors are noted in sufficient number, such as reversals,
rotations, and perseveration. Age, as expected, would also be
important and the test proves to be most useful for 7½ to
10-year-old children. The number of errors for the average 6-year-
old is 5, whereas the average numbers of errors for the 11-year-old is
1. Significant errors are only perceived as important after the child
has reached the chronological and mental age of 7 or 8 years. Again,
as with the WISC-R, the psychologist views the results on this test

with the understanding that experiential background and other variables can significantly influence the results and interpretation. Silver and Hagin (1960) have shown that "poor readers" make more errors on the BVMGT than do able readers. But again the BVMGT is not used in isolation, nor are causal relationships assumed between reading skills and visual-motor perception. However, visual-motor/visual-perceptual deficits noted on the BVMGT may tell us something about the Myklebust (1962) visual dyslexias — what Boder (1970) calls dyseidetic dyslexias — those who have difficulty in seeing whole words as gestalts. These dyslexic readers have trouble distinguishing small words from each other, yet they may know all of the phonetic blends. Lowell (1964) sees a relationship between perceptual problems demonstrated on the BVMGT and poor reading. Others have shown significant and substantial correlations (.51) between reading problems and reversals or rotations on this and other copying from model design tests. There is conflicting evidence in more recent studies, and Vellutino (1979) takes a critical view of clear relationships between pencil-paper/perceptual-motor tasks and reading difficulties. He seems to support Mercer (1979) in her contention that experience and sociocultural factors have significant effects on both reading and "grapho-motor" functions. There is no disputing this claim. However, a child with an enriched experiential background from the modal sociocultural group, who has average or above intelligence and shows a reversal rotation pattern on the BVMGT or the Beery-Buktenica VMI Test (1967) would be more suspect of being dyslexic if he or she were having "reading problems." Furthermore, from Boder's point of view, that child might be viewed as a dyseidetic dyslexic or possibly as a mixed dyslexic having both auditory and visual perceptual difficulties (dysphonetic-dyseidetic dyslexia).

Today, most psychologists also try to secure a writing sample during their assessments, particularly if one is not available from the educational assessment. Dysgraphia is frequently found in consort with dyslexia. Spelling problems also effect writing, particularly for the dysphonetic readers. As with other assessment instruments, some norm is necessary to evaluate this skill developmentally. At present there are instruments being investigated and standardized to do this. However, clinical judgment remains the method of analysis. The value of a writing sample is that it enables the examiner to check out and possibly validate hypotheses formed from other clinical data sources. It helps determine, by analysis of errors, the child's ability to transfer skills from one process to another and also may help determine the scope and magnitude of the handicap. It can assist in determining if the child has learned to compensate for reversal or rotation problems. Cicci (1980) cautions remedial teachers about focusing on only one segment of the reading-writing problems: "Just as a reading problem will affect the child's spelling, it will affect his having words available to use in longer units of written language. A child with a reading (and writing) problem needs remediation that combines work with reading, spelling and written formulation." The writing sample may also provide invaluable information on the discrepancy between the child's spoken language and written language. The child's approach to the task also helps the astute clinician determine how the child copes with school-like tasks and how frustration might be dealt with. One psychologist related a story about a 9-year-old child who was asked to write about a picture. The child immediately asked to go to the bathroom, then later he needed to sharpen his pencil, then requested paper without watermarks and finally after 15 minutes said, "You don't want to see my writing! No one can read it!" The child could not read the 15-word sample after it was painfully produced. This intelligent child was mildly dyslexic and severely dysgraphic and possibly on his way to becoming emotionally damaged.

When personality traits and emotional problems appear to cause the learning problem, there is a general tendency for the problem to be more global, affecting all areas that involve productivity. However, specific problems in reading can be the product of an emotional disturbance that may have a phobic quality to it or that may be associated with resentment or fear of growing up or with resistance to authority figures, parents or parent surrogates, or extreme feelings of worthlessness steming from a poor self-concept or depression. Sorting out this puzzle is part of the reason for examining emotional status. Here again the psychologist looks carefully at the environmental influences and frequently seeks out detailed information from parents, teachers, and other observers of the child. These materials move us away from the standardized, normed, referenced materials mentioned previously and move us toward the subjective and projective assessment tools that attempt to provide information into the undercurrents for the child's behavior.

Projective techniques are materials that are unstructured, relatively ambiguous, and have no right or wrong answers. They are interpreted by psychologists who recognize that the "tests" provide information about thought processes and personality dynamics that need to be validated.

Again we will provide a sample of the commonly used techniques, keeping in mind that there are hundreds of tests and techniques of merit which are simply not noted because they are less frequently administered when dealing with reading disabilities. The Rorschach-Inkblot Technique, the Thematic Apperception Test (TAT), the Children's Apperception Test (CAT), and Tasks of Emotional Development (TED) are frequently used projective techniques. There are also a variety of human figure drawing tasks which are viewed as projective, as well as developmentally perceptual-motor tasks, including the Draw-A-Person, the House-Tree-Person, and Kinetic family Drawing. In recent years checklists and rating scales have become popular along with word association and sentence completion tasks.

The Rorschach, which receives its name from its author, Hermann Rorschach, a Swiss psychiatrist, is the oldest of these techniques and the most studied. It is composed of 10 inkblots, some black and white and some multi-colored. The child is asked to tell what he sees in the blot. The responses are viewed in terms of their structure, content, the sequence, and use of elements of the blot. There are a variety of scoring systems used to analyze the responses, but they all deal with the concept of unconscious processes as they relate to adaption and to control of impulses and needs. Poor reality testing, phobic preoccupation, and depression and obsessional problems are substantiated by response analysis. With children, the response pattern must be viewed in terms of age-appropriate usual response patterns. Young children, for example, have a minimum number of responses since they have difficulty seeing two or more different responses to the same blot. Perseveration of responses and figure-ground reversals may suggest neurological problems that warrant further investigation.

The Thematic Apperception Test (TAT) and other picture story tests require the child to tell a story using the picture as the starting point. The TAT, CAT, and TED are less ambiguous than the Rorschach, and the TED is most specific to the child's environment being made up of photographs of children in a series of interactions with parents, siblings, and peers. The child tells a story in the present, past, and future. The identified leading character in the story is generally perceived to be a projection of the child who is telling the story. The TAT analysis focuses on needs and pressures within the child's interpersonal environment and the conflicts that may interfere with normal adaption. The CAT is based more directly upon the psychoanalytic theory of development. The TED is the most psychosocial of the three and focuses more strongly on the parent—peer—child relationships and self-concept in relation to these interactions. All three techniques are useful for assisting the psychologist in securing more information about the child's self-concept, defense mechanisms, reaction to anxiety-producing stimuli and problem-solving skills. The CAT and TED are more appropriate for younger children with the CAT being the choice for preschool children. Some learning disabled children whose self-concept has been seriously damaged by the handicap may project this theme over and over in the stories they make up. Children with emotional problems sometimes tend toward magical solutions or interpretations that are dramatic distortions to what is pictured. Again the skilled and experienced clinician reviews these samples of behavior in careful balance with other data knowing that the impact of an erroneous conclusion can harm the child. In psychology, unlike in the medical orientation, identification and labeling of a problem is a process in which false negatives are tolerated better than false positives, that is, psychologists feel it is better to say a child is not handicapped and be wrong than to say a child is handicapped and be wrong, since the latter decision frequently involves treatment that may dramatically change the child's self-concept as well as others' reactions to the child.

We have focused on psychometric and psychodiagnostic techniques that tell us about suspected pathology or weaknesses. These same techniques also provide a variety of measures of a child's strengths, both cognitively and emotionally. These samples of behavior may provide key information about a child's thinking style that has not been recognized before. They provide information about strong modalities that need constant use and reinforcement by the teacher to assist the child in compensating for whatever problem exists.

The other elements of the psychological evaluation are frequently supplied by other professionals in the multidisciplinary team that will make the proper diagnosis and prescriptive plan for the reading disabled child. These elements include: comprehensive medical and developmental history of the child, genetic and familial information, prenatal and birth information, milestones, parental attitude and parental rating scales of activity, and attention and orientation of the child over the years. Clear and complete information about the child's vision and hearing must be provided as well as orthopaedic concerns about known brain trauma. Language information is important. If the psychologist is expected to correct for sociocultural difference, we must also have that information available for the psychologist. Reports from other informants who know the child and family can be appropriate.

Behavioral observations by a trained specialist, such as a special educator, social worker, or psychologist, should be made within the educational environment in which the child is expected to function, and the observer should be aware of the concerns reported in the referral. The observer must also be able to provide information on the setting as well as on the teaching techniques utilized making sure that poor teaching is not the reason for the child's perceived problem.

Observation checklists are available as are training techniques for observers. The child's cognitive learning style should be noted. Is the child reflective or impulsive? Kagan's (1965) work on cognitive style has shown that reading disabled children have a greater tendency to respond impulsively to a visual matching task than able readers who appear more reflective. Some have felt that the more reflective cognitive style is a function of internal verbal mediating skills, which may be lacking in the impulsive responder. Task orientation and attention are important to consider. The hyperactive child with minimal brain dysfunction may show significant attention problems. Activity level is also important. This includes those "nervous" movements and unconscious tappings frequently noted. Language factors are also important to note. Observing the child's difficulty with the mechanics of the academic tasks is imperative. Is the child a fluent or dysfluent reader? Does the child comprehend what is read when it is read fluently? Are there frequent substitutions, reversals, or rotations when the child reads? What is the child's approach to reading, word attack style, attitude, level of anxiety? How does the child function on academic tasks that do not involve reading? What are the child's strengths? These are just some of the elements that should be focused upon and that can assist the psychologist in executing an appropriate assessment of the suspected learning disabled child.

The educational assessment is sometimes included in the psychological evaluation, but there appears to be a trend toward this aspect of the assessment being done by an educational specialist, such as a certified reading diagnostician, a learning disability specialist, or a special education teacher. For some years, the Wide Range Achievement Test (WRAT) was the most popular achievement test administered by psychologists. This test is standardized for youngsters age 5 through adult in two forms. It involves ''reading'' recognition of letters and words, spelling (writing words from dictation), and arithmetic, which includes counting, reading numbers, solving oral problems, and written computation. The ''reading'' part of this test tells us nothing about comprehension and provides a minimal sample of behaviors for a young age group. The arithmetic subtest is seen as a good test of written computation skills, provided the child has been exposed to the type of presentation in the test. The primary problem with the WRAT is that it provides a minimal amount of information for refined diagnosis.

Another standardized measure of reading is the Woodcock Reading Mastery Test, which provides much more diagnostic information than the WRAT. The Woodcock Reading Mastery Test consist of five subtests: letter identification, word identification, word attack (phonics), word comprehension, and passage comprehension. The test has norms for the school-age population for each subtest, and reported reliability and validity. The test also has special norms for various socioeconomic groups. The Woodcock is more diagnostic than the WRAT but again provides little information for very young children. It should be supplemented with an oral reading test to assist the clinician in diagnosis of fluency problems. For younger children another measure should be used. The Peabody Individual Achievement Tests (PIAT) like the WRAT, test a variety of academic skills including arithmetic, word recognition, reading comprehension, spelling, and general information. It was designed as a screening test but like the Woodcock, it is standardized and reported to be reliable and valid. The PIAT provides passage comprehension but the responses rely on visual discrimination skills, since the child must select the correct response from a set of four (except for the general information subtest where the child responds orally). Again no oral reading subtest is provided to evaluate fluency. The Stanford Diagnostic Reading Test is also normed and standardized being reliable and valid. It provides literal and inferential examples of comprehension which many other measures do not. Criterion referenced tests should also be administered to assist in establishing prescriptive goals and to clinically refine diagnosis. The Brigance Diagnostic Inventories is an example of this type of test.

Written expression is also measured in the educational assessment. The Test of Written Language has been developed with reported reliability and validity for youngsters 8 to 14. It provides measurement of mechanical, conventional, cognitive and linguistic skills.

Some parents and teachers expect children to perform as well in reading as they do in arithmetic, jump rope, and in the sharing of ideas in a discussion. There is a lack of understanding in development of a child's skills as to the variance and as to the differences in skills, some that will persist for life, which may be why people of equal ability become writers and others engineers. Some parents and teachers also assume that all children are average in their cognitive ability, which is not the case. Children in the *low average* IQ range are not expected to function at the same level as their *average* grade mates in reading. Expecting these children to read at this level will most probably produce frustration. In recent years an additional problem has occurred in our test-oriented, achievement-oriented society and that is that a child with a *Superior* IQ is expected to read, write sentences and do math at a superior level. However, all of the research and statistical techniques tell us that, when one is predicting achievement from intelligence (correlated measures) the predicted value will, on the average, regress toward the mean (McLeod, 1979). Children with IQs lower than the mean of 100 will have achievement standard scores that are closer to 100 than their IQ would predict and children with higher IQs than average will have achievement scores that are lower and closer to average than their IQs would predict. Looking at the IQs in Table 3-3 the hypothesized regression effect on educational achievement can be seen.

Furthermore, when predicting academic achievement from intelligence quotients, the error factor is significant since both mea-

Table 3-3
IQ and Educational Quotient

IQ Score	Educational Quotient (EQ)
130 (Very Superior)	123.6
120–129 (Superior)	118.4
110–119 (High Average)	109.1
100–109 (Average)	103.0
90–99 (Average)	95.1
80–89 (Low Average)	89.6
70–79 (Borderline)	83.9
69 and below (Mentally Deficient)	Not Computed

(Modification of simulated data provided from McLeod, 1978, p. 325).

sures are affected by errors of measurement, which all the more emphasizes the need for good clinical analysis and cross-validated multiple samples of behavior.

For many years a dyslexic reader was viewed as one who had a normal or above average intelligence and who was reading two years below grade level. This concept has long been discarded. Many research projects and practical situations have demonstrated the futility of rigidly adhering to any arbitrary grade level definition, since it is obvious that as a child gets older, a two-grade level difference between expectancy and functioning becomes less meaningful. Conceptually, there is little difference between a grade 13 reading level and a grade 11 reading level. Furthermore, it has been discovered over and over again that grade-level measures are subject to the highest degree of error and vary significantly from one reading test to another, and, since intelligence quotients are age-based standard scores and grade levels are not, the two cannot be compared. Therefore, it is important to convert any reading scores to age equivalent scores and then, when possible, to standard scores so that they can be properly compared to IQs as noted in the above table.

Children who are having difficulty in school must be given careful psychological examinations directed at identifying their areas of strength and weakness. A good psychological report will contain concepts demonstrating that the search for key disorders was done in a comprehensive and systematic fashion, so that there is little likelihood of false positive or negative findings. This concept of searching through test channels to find both specific cognitive skills and specific areas of dysfunction is extremely important if one is to know how to systematize a treatment strategy for the child's improvement.

The teacher who does not understand about the connections and learning channels may commit many major errors in dealing with a child with a learning disability. For example, the teacher is likely to spend excessive time, even years, trying to develop a totally nonfunctioning auditory system. In the same child, the teacher may also spend an inordinate amount of time attempting to develop a kinesthetic system beyond the potential usefulness of that system. In pursuing these two aims in the child, the teacher runs a high risk of not fully utilizing other, more adequate channels of learning. If the child is functionally deaf, the auditory language may not be fully utilized. By persisting in working with the impossible learning areas, the teacher is likely to invoke in the child serious psychiatric influences, overtones, or background because of the constant frustration and failures that have been imposed upon the child.

Using the proper test channels during the diagnostic examination of a child suspected of a learning disability can reveal whether the child's disability is of peripheral or of central origin, and a complete psychological report can indicate which specific central factor is involved in the learning problem.

Mark (1969) has devised a chart in which there is a hierarchy of central nervous system functions of "systems" that emerge in normal development as an ordered set in each of the channels of communication. The emergence order of these systems is compatible with the norms for developmental milestones published by Gesell and coworkers in 1956 and by Terman and Merrill in 1960. They differ primarily from developmental milestones in that Mark subdivides the system within each channel into subsystems, subsubsystems, and so on, thereby permitting a more finely grained analysis of a child's learning strengths and weaknesses. Entering mental measurements on a subject into such a chart permits the tester to report systematicallly not only strengths and weaknesses, but also pseudostrengths ("halo effects") and pseudoweaknesses, which often obscure the real mental ability profile of the person. Furthermore, Mark's diagnostic search strategy is aimed at finding the most basic learning disability which can "account for" the largest number of secondary disabilities within the hierarchy of developmental milestones in each channel. These basic disabilities then automatically become the target of educational treatment and/or circumvention strategies.

After a proper evaluation there will be no wasted time and effort, which brings havoc into the emotional well-being of the child and his family. Rather, by examination of these individual areas of learning skills, one can acquire an adequate learning disability profile. From this profile, proper teaching techniques and strategies can be developed for the individual student.

The psychological evaluation, therefore, provides a means of indicating which children should be identified as either developmental readers, corrective readers, or remedial readers. With regard to the latter two groups, the analysis should give an indication of the best steps to take toward correction or remediation of the problem. For the severely learning disabled reader, the psychological evaluation should result in specific recommendations regarding changes in the psychoeducational environment of the individual child that may enable him to achieve adequate reading skills. The range of possible psychoeducational modifications is quite broad, and the specific changes recommended will depend upon the nature of each child's learning disability.

REFERENCES

Bannatyne, A. Diagnosis: A note on recategorization of the WISC scaled scores. *Journal of Learning Disabilities,* 1974, *7,* 272–274.

Bannatyne, A. *Language, reading aand learning disabilities.* Springfield, Illinois: Charles C. Thomas Publishers, 1971.

Beery, K. and Buktenica, N. *Developmental test of visual-motor integration.* Chicago: Follett, 1967.

Bender, L. A Visual Motor Gestalt Test and its clinical use. *Research Monographs of the American Orthopsychiatric Association,* 1938, No. 3.

Birch, H. Dyslexia and maturation of visual function. In J. Money (ed.) *Reading disability: Progress and research needs in dyslexia.* Baltimore, Maryland: John Hopkins Press, 1962.

Boder, E. Developmental dyslexia: A diagnostic approach based on the identification of three subtypes. *Journal of School Health,* 1970, *40,* 289–290.

Burgemeister, B. B., Blum, L. H., and Lorge, I. *Columbia mental maturity scale (3 ed.).* New York: Harcourt Brace Jovanovich, 1972.

Campbell, P. Study links learning disabilities with delinquency. *ETS Developments*. Princeton, New Jersey: Educational Testing Service, 1979, (2), 21–22.

Cicci, R. Written language disorders. *Bulletin of the Orton Society,* 1980, *30,* 240–251.

Dunn, L. M. *Peabody picture vocabulary test: Manual of directions and norms.* Nashville, Tennessee: American Guidance Service, 1959.

Dwyer, K. Learning disabilities and language disabilities: Can a multidisciplinary team approach to diagnosis and planning help? Unpublished presentation, CEC Convention, New York, April 14, 1981.

Gesell, A., Ilg, F., and Anes. L. *Youth: The years from ten to sixteen.* New York: Harper and Row, 1956.

Goh, D., Teslow, C., and Fuller, G. Psychological test usage among school psychologists. Unpublished presented at National Association of School Psychologists Annual Convention, Washington, D.C., April 10, 1980.

Jansky, J., and DeHirsch, K. *Preventing reading failure: Prediction, diagnosis, intervention.* New York: Harper and Row, 1972.

Kagan, J. Reflection-impulsivity and reading ability in primary grade children. *Child Development,* 1965, *36,* 609–628.

Kaufman, A. A new approach to the interpretation of test scatter on the WISC-R. *Journal of Learning Disabilities,* 1976, *9,* 160–168.

Kaufman, A. Factor analysis of the WISC-R at eleven age levels between 6½ and 16½ years. *Journal of Consulting and Clinical Psychology,* 1975, *43,* 135–147.

Kaufman, A. *Intelligent testing with the WISC-R.* New York: Wiley-Interscience, 1979.

Kaufman, A. The WISC-R and LD assessment: State of the art. *Journal of Learning disabilities* (in press).

Koppitz, E. *The Bender-Gestalt test for young children.* New York: Grune and Stratton, Inc., 1964.

Lambert, N. School psychology training for the decades ahead or rivers, streams and creeks: Currents and tributaries to the sea. *School Psychology Review,* Spring, 1981, *10* (2), 194–205.

Lowell, K., and Oliver, P. A study of some cognitive and other disabilities in backward readers of average non-verbal reasoning scores. *British Journal of Educational Psychology,* 1964, *34,* 275–279.

Mark, H. Psychodiagnostics in patients with suspected minimal brain dysfunction: Minimal brain dysfunction. HEW Monograph, Washington, D.C.: U.S. Dept. of Health, Education, and Welfare, PHS-2015, 1969.

McLeod, J. Educational underachievement: Toward a defensible psychometric definition. *Journal of Learning Disabilities,* 1979, *12,* 322–330.

McLeod, J. *Psychometric identification of children with learning disabilities*. Saskatoon, Canada: University of Saskatchewan, Institute of Child Guidance and Development, 1978.

Mercer, J. R. *SOMPA: System of Multicultural Pluralistic Assessment: Technical Manual*. New York: The Psychological Corporation, 1979.

Myklebust, H., and Johnson, D. Dyslexia in children. *Exceptional Children,* 1962, *29,* 14–25.

Rugel, R. WISC subtest scores of disabled readers: A review *Journal of Learning Disabilities,* 1974, *7,* 48–55.

Silver, A., and Hagin, R. Specific reading disability: Delineation of the syndrome and relationship to cerebral dominance. *Comparative Psychiatry,* 1960, *1* (2), 126–134.

Slosson, R. *Slosson intelligence test*. East Aurora, New York: Slosson Educational Publications, 1971.

Stark, J. Collaborative planning for the student with a learning disability: The language perspective. Unpublished presentation, CEC Convention, New York, April 14, 1981.

Terman, L. and Merrill, M. *Stanford-Binet intelligence scale (1972 norms edition)*. Boston: Houghton, Mifflin, 1973.

Vellutino, F. *Dyslexia: Theory and research*. Cambridge, Massachusetts: MIT Press, 1979.

Wechsler, D. *WPPSI Manual–Wechsler preschool and primary scales of intelligence*. New York: The Psychological Corporation, 1967.

Wechsler, D. *WISC-R Manual–Wechsler intelligence scales for children-revised*. New York: The Psychological Corporation, 1974.

4

Neurological Aspects

In many instances the very medical advances that have saved the lives of children have also increased the number of children with disabilities. The phenomenon of brain damage in children offers a striking example of these advances. Many children who formerly would have died at birth survive today due to antibiotic treatment and other life-saving techniques. Research information and services are becoming increasingly available and identification and diagnosis are readily made. There are many children, however, whose brain damage is less obvious and whose manifestations are characterized by "soft signs," of which "perceptual deficit" is one example. These children are frequently overlooked in the educational system and often misunderstood and labeled "problem children" by their perplexed parents and teachers.

The child whose reading problem results from brain damage is the most difficult to diagnose. Even when minimal brain damage or cerebral dysfunction is present, the child may appear to be completely normal. A physical examination will frequently not show anything abnormal, and intelligence tests may show scores in the average or above average range. A sizable number of children with superior intelligence have reading difficulties because of some degree of brain dysfunction that does not reveal itself in any consistent manner.

It is important that physicians and teachers recognize the symptoms of such dysfunction in handicapped readers. When the

41

child suffers an insult to the central nervous system, either prenatally, perinatally, or postnatally, it may impose a severe threat to the integrity of the child's emotional system.

Rappaport (1965) and others have reported major areas of difficulty in children who have suffered an insult to the central nervous system, manifested in problems of perception and concept formation. There are children who appreciate a stimulus but who have trouble relating it to everyday situations. These children can acquire many facts but sometimes have great difficulty applying such information to functional situations. The major problem is in concept formation. The child can work with the concrete and specific but has difficulty with the abstract.

A second problem area these children experience is a lack of adequate impulse control. These children are often hyperactive and distractible. Some of the symptoms may be due to lack of neural control, but they can also be a defense against emotional instability.

A third area of concern for the brain-injured child involves their emotional defense mechanisms. Children who have had an early insult to the central nervous system often feel apprehensive and anxious. They may become aggressive or withdrawn and may retreat from learning situations because further failure represents a severe threat to their self-esteem.

In some cases, the effects of such damage may not be evidenced except in the child's inability to interpret written material or to associate concepts with symbols.

From 1915 to 1921 an epidemic of encephalitis—sleeping sickness—swept the world. The disease, which causes edema in the brain, drew a great amount of attention. These cases were described lucidly by Ford (1966).

There is in most cases no marked reduction of intelligence, but personality changes of a profound nature frequently result. In most cases, physical signs are absent or trivial. These children are very destructive and impulsive. Any impulse which occurs to them is at once translated into action. Their misdeeds are not planned, but are the result of the temptation of the moment. The natural inhibitions of fear of consequence, which restrain all of us from injudicious behavior, seem to be lacking in these children. Without any thought of punishment, they will steal, lie, destroy property, set fires and commit various offenses. They usually make no effort to evade detection, and when reproached with their conduct, will reply that they could not help it. They may be quite indifferent to punishment, or may exhibit exaggerated remorse for their offense, which, however, does not prevent further misdeeds. An important factor in these behavior disorders is the emotional instability. The child's mood changes in response to the slightest stimulus. Most patients are very restless and overactive, hurrying from one form of mischief to another throughout the day. The children often run away from home and are impatient of any restraint. This is the neurological background in which these children must learn.

There have been occasional reports, one as early as 1892, of the postmortem examination of the brain of a person who had suffered from alexia. (Alexia is a condition wherein a person has lost previous ability to read and to recognize letters of words, and yet is still able to write spontaneously. Alexia is similar to the word dyslexia, but dyslexia is usually reserved to describe those who have "word blindness" from birth.) In 1892, Dejerine published a case of a patient who, after having had a cerebrovascular accident (stroke) developed an inability to read. He identified this inability as alexia. A number of years later, this patient died of a major stroke. The postmortem examination of his brain revealed a lesion in the subcortical region of the left angular gyrus, suggesting that a lesion in the left angular gyrus might have accounted for inability to read.

Similarly, children who have brain damage may demonstrate neurological signs that are referable to the parietal lobes. Such lesions in the parietal lobes of the dominant and nondominant hemispheres can each reveal findings that are compatible with signs frequently found in dyslexia.

Lesions in the dominant parietal lobe are suggested by dysgraphia, dyscalculia, finger agnosia, errors in right—left discrimination, dyspraxia, and even dyslexia. Dysfunction in the nondominant parietal lobe is suggested by disorders of body image, unilateral spatial imperception, spatial agnosia, and constructional apraxia. There may be overt signs of damage or injury that a careful neurological examination can, on occasion, reveal to the pediatric neurologist. Most frequently, however, there are no obvious signs of damage, and this leads to the application of the term "cerebral dysfunction." In essence, the signs are just too minimal to be identified with neurological impairment although the following characteristics are present:

1. Intelligence, as formally measured, is within the average range or only moderately reduced, although more careful scrutiny of subtests brings out some significant observations. Intelligence

may be low for the expected average for the family, and the scatter within intelligence tests may be remarkably wide. Tests involving rote memory are generally best performed, while those involving step-by-step reasoning from premise to premise, and those involving perception of spatial and form relationships, are done very poorly.

2. Physical signs of neurological abnormality are absent or trivial. Minor inequalities of reflexes, slight asymmetries of development, an occasional extensor plantar response, may be all that is seen. If one looks carefully, a real profusion of signs and symptoms can often be distinguished. Children with learning disabilities are quite often moderately delayed in attaining physical milestones of development, particularly those requiring fine motor control. Sitting, walking, and the like may not be much delayed (if at all), but handedness, normally clearly foreshadowed by 18 to 24 months, is usually delayed to the fourth or fifth year. The child may run about freely, but does not have the ability to ride a bicycle for years, and fastening buttons may be impossible until the child is 6 or 7 years old. Clear-cut apraxia is seldom present, but an effort to tie his shoelaces brings out frantic turnings and twistings; and hopping on one foot, a task the normal five year old does well, is clumsy and unsteady.

3. Emotional instability is evidenced. These children swing from violent aggressiveness, through extreme timidity, clinging to the parents, with effusive emotionality, and then back to tears— almost as they are being watched. This is combined with another feature: a marked hyperactivity and distractability. These are the children who have tremendous difficulty sitting still, who are constantly on the go, roaming about the consulting room, peering into drawers, running to the window at every sound, poking into one's pockets, climbing onto a chair, or refusing to be touched. Their physical awkwardness and unpredictable mood swing make it hard for these children to find friends, and the parents almost always recount that either they have no friends at all, not infrequently because the neighbors have forbidden their own children to associate with the neighborhood outcast, or else that they play with a much younger child.

When the parents are asked to describe what exactly the child does that is so "bad," they usually are at a loss to think of anything of any significance. In the words of one parent, "It is not that his behavior is so bad, it is just that there is so much of it." Questioned more closely, the mother will generally agree that when the child is alone with her, he can perform quite well and is often quiet and lovable, although, even then, hyperactive and distractible to a degree. His schoolwork is poor, and he gets good marks only in those things he can, in one way or another, commit to memory.

Efforts to tutor him are usually poor, especially if it involves keeping him working at one task for more than 20 minutes.

Other difficulties may be present, the most common ones having to do with the child's development of speech and language. These vary from slow development of infantile articulation, difficulties and substitutions in the use of connecting words and phrases, to outright aphasias. Reading difficulties often result from frequent failures to recognize and distinguish between various words and forms, as well as from reversals and a marked difficulty with perception of shape, form, and spatial relationships. School children of 8 or 9 years old may have no grasp of the spatial arrangement of the words in a sentence and be quite unable to copy simple geometric forms from memory, even with the originals before them.

As noted, the physical examination of such children is unrevealing until one begins to search for the evidences of early aphasia and apraxia, by tests of shoelace tying, figure copying, hopping, copying of dictated material, and the like. Laboratory examinations also may not be helpful.

To understand the complicated process of reading and the effect brain damage may have upon it, we must understand the parts and areas of the brain which becomes involved in the reading process.

First, the printed word is seen by the eye, which serves only to form an image which is relayed to the brain for interpretation. These images are transmitted as electrical impulses from the retina of the eye to the optic nerve, and then to the occipital cortex, known as Brodmann's area 17. This area is the first to receive the visual signal. Injury to this part of the brain may produce slow reading because of the inability to identify the written word. Area 18 in the brain is next to area 17 and surrounds it like a reversed letter C. This area is activated only by impulses starting in area 17 and is concerned only with visual memory patterns. It is this area which enables children to see objects such as a chair or a cat and to remember the visual images so that they recognize them the next time they see them. The upper part of area 18 functions in the recognition of animate objects, such as the cat, while the lower part acts in the recognition of inanimate objects, such as the chair. Destruction of this area results in loss of ability to recognize objects and is called visual agnosia. The ability to read, however, is not usually affected.

Area 19, also shaped like the letter C, surrounds area 18, and is stimulated by area 18. It is concerned with the elaboration of memory patterns necessary for the recall of animate and inanimate objects and also of language symbols. Destruction of this area results in loss of memory of things, of persons, and of language. A patient may not be able to tell the difference between an apple and an orange nor be able to read.

Another area of the brain that is essential in both the reading and writing process is called the angular gyrus. Injury to the angular gyrus will cause a person to be unable to read. In this instance, the individual sees the printed word but cannot interpret it.

An area known as Wernicke's area is concerned with the recognition and recall of speech. Since there are nerve connections between Wernicke's area and the angular gyrus, and since this area reinforces the ability to understand written language by auditory stimulation or by hearing the word, this area comes into play in the learning process (e.g., when the teacher speaks a word and ask the child to repeat what is heard).

A final area of the brain that is of importance in the learning process is the area of Broca, which is also connected with the angular gyrus and is concerned with the motor function of speech. Its function is demonstrated by those individuals whose silent reading is associated with lip movement. In these cases the visual image stimulates the muscles that have to do with speaking, demonstrating the close connection between the visual and speech areas of the brain.

Injury in either Wernicke's area or Broca's area can complicate the learning process (especially when the teacher uses classroom techniques that involve hearing the spoken word and repeating what is heard).

If there is a lesion in the left occipital lobe and another lesion in the splenium of the corpus collosum, no impulses from the primary visual areas can reach the left angular gyrus. The person thus affected suffers from alexia without agraphia (agraphia meaning the inability to write). So, alexia without agraphia occurs when there is a lesion in the angular gyrus of the left cerebral hemisphere. Alexia alone occurs when there is a lesion in the angular gyrus plus a lesion in the corpus collosum.

Children who suffer from dyslexia may be able to recognize letters if they trace them with their finger. This is because the impulses originating in the parietal cortex of the brain, which bring kinesthetic information from the tracing finger, are sent to the angular gyrus where decoding impulses of visual, auditory, and kinesthetic origin have been encoded and previously memorized. Therefore, the reading disabled child may have lost the ability to recognize words or letters, but can still see and write spontaneously.

Perception and visual interpretation is another important part of reading. This involves the Gestalt phenomenon and consists of a putting together of the visual impulses. Figure 4-1 is a series of dots, which the normal brain does not perceive as being isolated, but rather as being a square and a triangle sitting on a line. Thus the brain perceives these dots as an organized configuration.

Figure 4-2 shows another series of dots. This one is more complex. Here, the normal brain will perceive the grouping of shapes as a man on horseback, possibly with some action indicated. In this case, a person who has brain damage may not perceive the horse.

In this way the brain builds up a visual pattern. This Gestalt phenomenon is also illustrated in reading. If children with visual-motor disability or incoordination see the teacher flash a word, they may not be able to see it as a complete word but only as a series of letters without meaning.

Historically, brain dysfunction has been suspected of being a cause of learning disabilities, and in 1947 Strauss and Lehtinen wrote one of the first books on the psychopathology and education of the brain injured child, stressing the psychological drawings of children suspected of brain damage.

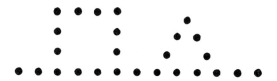

Figure 4-1. Perceptual configuration: A square and a triangle.

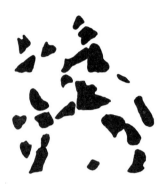

Figure 4-2. Perceptual configuration: Man on horseback.

Kawi and Pasamanik (1958) reviewed the records of 205 children who had reading problems and found that 16.9 percent of them had been exposed to two or more complications during birth or immediately thereafter. Records of a control group of children without reading problems revealed that only 1.5 percent of this group had complications at birth.

Kawi and Pasamanik concluded that the complications encountered by these children at birth were such that they may have caused some degree of lowered oxygen content to the brain (fetal anoxia). Since the blood vessels to the brain are terminal or end vessels, these areas are the first to be affected by a lack of oxygen. They reported that severe cases of fetal anoxia result in miscarriage, stillbirth, spontaneous abortion, and neonatal death. Less serious forms of oxygen deprivation may result in cerebral palsy and epilepsy, while very minor injury leads to behavior problems, speech disorders, and delayed reading. This report was one of the first indications in modern research that indicated there was a neurological condition associated with dyslexia or learning disability.

In his writings on the development of children, Gesell (1967) noted that unrecognized minimal birth injury may express itself in speech difficulty and may appear later in the form of reading difficulty. When observing such children. Gesell noticed they were clumsy: they could not button their shirts, had poor hand–eye coordination when bouncing a ball, and showed general lack of muscular coordination.

A "continuum" suggested by Kawi and Pasamanik (1958) that outlines an ordinary progression of severity of involvement of the central nervous system due to anoxia appears supportable. In dyslexia, the changes are minimal and may exist with no manifest organic lesion. The changes result from altered molecular protein synthesis. So the relationship of brain damage to prematurity does exist, but the implication of prematurity to learning disabilities does not necessarily follow. Also, the greater the frequency of ocular findings in cerebral palsy, the more severe is the mental retardation (Landau and Berson, 1971). Similarly, the less severe the mental retardation, the less severe the accompanying ocular defects. Therefore, the more extreme the prematurity, the more severe the brain damage, and the less extreme the prematurity, the less severe the brain damage.

In addition to the study of Kawi and Pasamanik (1958) a report was published by Walsh and Lindenberg (1961) that demonstrated the damage to optic nerve pathways that occurred when the child suffered from hypoxia, or lack of oxygen. Agreeing with Kawi and Pasamanik, they contended that children could suffer from varying degrees of hypoxia and perinatal distress. Both groups concluded that if there was a considerable oxygen lack, then spontaneous abortion or stillborn birth could occur. With less severe degrees of oxygen lack, the child would perhaps suffer from epilepsy or cerebral palsy; and with minimal degrees of hypoxia or oxygen lack, a less severe neurological impairment could result in the child developing speech difficulties or learning disabilities. This anoxia was similarly responsible for involvement of the optic pathways.

Other research soon demonstrated the possibility of neurological handicaps in another way. This is associated with the finding that some children cannot reproduce geometric designs or do tasks such as drawing a box, a triangle, or a flag. This finding coincides with Bender-Gestalt Test findings which often reveal that children with brain damage may have an inability to reproduce meaningful geometric forms. This difficulty in drawing geometric forms, and the inability to perform successfully the Bender-Gestalt Test, is further evidence of cerebral dysfunction and has become a symptom complex associated with soft neurological signs. Richmond Payne (1962) discussed the minimal chronic brain syndrome in children, while Prechtyl and Stemmer (1962) emphasized the prominence of choreiform movements (a wide variety of rapid, jerky but well-coordinated and involuntary movements) as a symptom of minimal brain damage.

Among diagnostic procedures, the psychological tests are of great value. A well-explained WISC-R (see Chapter 3) will contribute to our understanding of a reading disability, especially if the child demonstrates subtest scatter. Frequently, it is the performance scale of the WISC-R that is most significant and most affected in neurological dysfunction.

The diagnosis of possible brain damage can be reinforced by a careful perinatal history of the child. The mother may have had some complications of pregnancy before or during birth, perhaps a convulsive seizure, a hypotensive episode, or exposure to drugs, tobacco, or alcohol. Postnatal brain damage might have resulted from dehydration or head injury. Perhaps there was a high bilirubin level at birth, or there may have been low birth weight.

Tests of perception may provide our most positive evidence for making a diagnosis of minimal brain dysfunction. There are a number of tests which are helpful, including those of matching geometric designs and the figure–ground discrimination test.

In 1964, Birch and Belmont devised a test which involved the matching of Morse Code signals to printed dots or dot-dash combinations. This is a test of short-term memory. Another test of immediate memory involves digit repetition, or the ability of the child to repeat sequences of numbers backward and forward. This ability is often quite poor in children who have minimal brain dysfunction but who, by contrast, may also have a good memory for facts or the ability to memorize in general. Obviously, both attention and motivation affect the results of these types of tests.

Also, in the minimal brain dysfunction group, a test of praxia frequently will reveal some impairment. This involves the drawing of a geometric design from memory or the ability to place furniture or reproduce a floor plan of a familiar room.

A frequent sign of possible organic dysfunction is the child's inability to button his shirt or to tie his shoes. In some cases of minimal brain dysfunction, there is an impairment of the ability to perceive figures traced on the skin with a blunt instrument (graphaesthesia).

Other evidence of neurological involvement was explained in the work of Khoudadoust (1968) who studied 1,000 children who had been born at a hospital in Baltimore, Maryland. He took pictures of the retina (fundus photography) and found that 25 percent of these children had evidence of retinal hemorrhages (see Figure 4-3). A

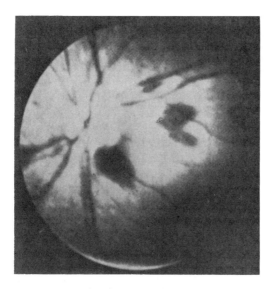

Figure 4-3. Retinal hemorrhages in newborn infant in the first 48 hours of life.

survey of existing literature revealed three other medical studies which also reported a 25 percent incidence of hemorrhages in the retina of the newborn. Analysis of these figures suggested that if the mother had had no previous children (primipara), there was a 39 percent chance of the child having retinal hemorrhages. If, however, the mother was multiparous (having had children before), the frequency of retinal hemorrhages dropped to approximately 21 percent. In other words, there is evidence of retinal hemorrhages in newborn children, and these findings suggest that there is a possibility that some damage may be done to the child's central nervous system at birth as the child passes through the birth canal. Since head circumference of the male is larger than the female, it is probable and understandable that retinal hemorrhages and birth injury in the male is more frequent than in the female. Other evidence of birth damage lies in electroencephalographic changes.

Double-blind brain wave studies were performed on 100 children (Goldberg et. al., 1960). Fifty of these children had severe degrees of reading disability but no overt signs of neurological damage. When the EEG tracings of a control group of 50 normal children were compared to this group, the children with severe reading disabilities registered a higher instance of EEG abnormalities.

At this point, it is important to understand what the electroencephalograph is and how it works. The brain sends out waves of energy, much the same as a radio or television transmitter, except that the brain waves are only by-products and, like smoke from a factory chimney, they give only a general indication of what is actually going on inside. For example, it is not possible to relate specific thoughts to specific EEG patterns. More recently positron emission transaxial tomography (PETT) seems to be able to accomplish the relationship of specific thoughts to specific patterns. By the injection of irradiated glucose, which is metabolized in the brain, x-rays can demonstrate the areas of the brain that are being used in relation to the specific thought process.

To begin, electrodes are placed on different parts of the head. They pick up the waves that are being transmitted from the particular parts of the brain nearest to them. These waves are amplified; and traced onto moving graph paper as a permanent record of the wave pattern. These patterns indicate if the brain is functioning normally or whether there is damage present in any particular area. A sudden discharge, wave slowing, or lack of wave activity from any area may indicate injury or disease.

Figure 4-4 shows such a graph, recorded from a person with normal wave activity. The lines are fairly regular in pattern. The normal rhythm is generally 8 to 13 cycles per second. The top four lines record the right side of the brain, and the lower four lines record the left hemisphere. (Numerous other combinations are possible.) When the recordings of a delayed reader are manifested, slowing and peaking of wave lengths results (see Figure 4-5).

Penfield (1959), a neurosurgeon, operated on 17 patients who had focal epilepsy as a result of brain damage involving the parieto-occipital area. They were given psychological and visual–motor tests, and also had routine brain wave tracings, both before and after the operation. The test results indicated that these children had suffered no impairment of intellectual capacity. The EEGs showed abnormalities such as we found with delayed readers, and visual–motor disturbances appeared which were the same as those found in other cases of delayed readers.

Electroencephalograms have been performed on reading disabled children before, but rarely with rigid conditions of testing.

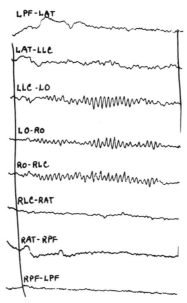

Figure 4-4. Normal EEG of a 12½ year old.

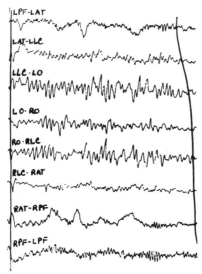

Figure 4-5. EEG demonstrating slowing and peaking in a delayed reader.

Kennard (1952), for example, performed EEGs on delayed readers who were in a psychiatric ward. She found abnormalities in nearly 80 percent of the cases, but it is well known that the brain wave tracing may be abnormal if a patient is in a psychotic state. In itself, the EEG is not diagnostic and must never be considered alone but only as one of many findings. Even then its findings are not always conclusive.

Many cases could be cited which show the similarities between reactions of children with known brain damage and those children identified as disabled readers. The question we must ask now is, "what causes such brain dysfunction?" Unfortunately, no one has the exact answer as the brain is extremely complicated and much about its functioning still remains unknown.

Thus far we have mentioned positive EEG findings, the failure to do geometric drawings, the studies of Kawi and Pasamanik (1958) and the studies of Walsh and Lindenberg (1961)—all of which have suggested strong evidence for the presence of cerebral dysfunction. Other investigations have been conducted that are even stronger in their indication of the presence of possible brain dysfunction as a cause of learning disabilities.

Towbin (1971) found cerebral and cortical damage in children who had varying degrees of hypoxia and actually demonstrated histological evidence of cortical atrophy. This information, when combined with the previous studies noted previously, provide evidence that damage to the brain, either major or minimal, chemical or enzymatic, can produce a dysfunction that could result in a learning disability.

With reference to the early detection of neurological abnormalities in newborn infants, serum bilirubin levels and low birth weight are important indicators. Routinely studying the bilirubin levels of a large number of newborns, Hardy and Peeples (1971) found that 84 percent had maximum levels below 10 milligrams; 5 percent had bilirubin levels of 15 milligrams or above, and 2 percent had levels of 20 milligrams or more. They also noted that babies weighing 1500 grams or less, and those born after less than 37 weeks of gestation, had significantly higher levels of serum bilirubin than the larger, more mature infants. Comparisons made between control groups of full-term infants have indicated that there are significantly more deaths in the neonatal period in children with high bilirubin levels than among control groups. There also may be significant differences in the intelligence levels of the two groups.

The maturing brain, both before and after birth, may suffer damage that ultimately results in an impairment of neurologic function. This damage may result not only in poorer functioning of the central nervous system but also in an aberration of function.

The cause of minimal brain dysfunction has been linked to environmental influences, heredity, nutrition, toxicity, endocrine, and other processes. Birch's (1964) review of the various problems related to brain damage in children pointed out that brain damage can vary with respect to many factors. These include: origin, extent, location, type of lesion, duration of damage, the rate at which the damage has been sustained and the time of life or developmental stage at which the injury has occurred.

The relationship of learning disability to brain damage is still received with caution by some and skepticism by others. Based upon the results of studies on perinatal histories, psychological testing and drawings, EEG tracings, and frequent evidence of retinal hemorrhages in the newborn, it may be concluded that there is a percentage of children with minimal brain dysfunction who are learning disabled.

Towbin (1971) has been able to study neuropathological material and has collected over 600 neonatal case studies. He has demonstrated that four main forms of cortical and spinal damage occur in the human fetus and the newborn. These four forms are (1) subdural hemorrhage caused by traumatic dural venous tears; (2) spinal cord and brain stem damage caused by mechanical injury at birth; (3) anoxic damage to the deep cerebral structures, which occurs mainly in the premature child; and (4) hypoxic damage to the cerebral cortex in the mature fetus and the newborn child. Any resulting injury depends upon two factors: (1) the severity of the episode of oxygen lack, and (2) the location of the lesion in the brain.

Pathologically, Towbin found two consistent factors. Some of the lesions showed persistent hemosiderin, which is the consequence of a previous hemorrhage, and others demonstrated glial scarring. He also identified another type of lesion which he termed ischemic neuronal necrosis. In this condition there was an ultimate decrease of neurons in the brain. This decrease could account for inhibition or distortion of proper brain function. The decrease of neurons was so lightly distributed that it escaped detection even when the tissue was examined microscopically. A loss of up to 30 percent of cells may be unrecognized even by an experienced neuropathologist. This type of loss of cellular elements of the brain, although not visible anatomically, may be associated with specific learning disability in a child.

In the period from 1960 to 1970, there was a great tendency for those involved in the learning disability field to indiscriminately use the label "brain damage." This label was unfortunate in that it created a sense of apprehension and despair in both parents and teachers. Eventually, this diagnostic term was droped from the educator's vocabulary. A host of other names were then applied to the problem, including minimal cerebral dysfunction, chronic brain dysfunction or syndrome, or minimal brain dysfunction—all synonymous with "brain damage." "Minimal cerebral dysfunction" was perhaps the least objectionable term because it lacked the words "damaged" or "injured." It is important to note that these latter two words often implied to parents a situation of futility, and possibly diminished some teachers' motivation to teach the child.

It is very important to understand that children who fulfilled the criteria of minimal brain damage at an early age may not be truly brain damaged. For example, there is a group of children historically known as immature or "late bloomers." These are children who exhibit some immaturity until 8 years of age. Not every child who begins school at the age of 5 or 6 is actually ready for school.

It is also very important that there be communication between parents and teachers, especially when a child has a specific learning disability where brain damage is a possible etiological factor. Teachers must be made aware of the fact that it is their responsibility to teach no matter what the origin or severity of the reading problem might be. Often children have attributes and capabilities equal to or far beyond their years. If they can be discovered, attention should be directed toward these areas of proficiency.

The evidence for immaturity may be drawn from different diagnostic sources. For example, on the "Draw-A-Person" test, there is an observable maturational lag in the immature child's drawings. Another significant finding lies in x-rays, which when taken of the small bones of the hands and feet (the metacarpals and metatarsals) tend to demonstrate ossification at a much earlier age in the female than in the male. For instance, in a 6-year-old girl there is a 2 year difference in the ossification of the greater multiangular wrist bone than that of a 6-year-old boy. This immaturity provides another reason for greater incidence of learning disability in the male as compared to the female. Maturational differences such as this account in some way for the reading readiness of some and the lack of readiness of others at the same age.

To call these children "brain damaged" would be erroneous. If they are recognized, and properly taught, these "immature children" can succeed (and could even be superior) at a later age.

Parents also constitute a part of the problem of managing children with brain dysfunction especially since many of them have difficulty accepting the fact that their children do have some type of disability. As a result, our society is full of parents who are overzealously involved in the field of learning disabilities because their children have a problem which, when it involves reading, is usually defined by the parents as "dyslexia." This word is often easier and less stigmatic for a parent to accept than the term "brain damaged."

From the medical point of view, the management of those children who have a specific learning disability due to brain damage is rather limited. Certainly acute intoxication, such as lead poisoning, should be eliminated. Also, metabolic diseases should be diagnosed and controlled, and of these the phenylketonuria (PKU) and aminoacidurias in some atypical form must be considered. Intracranial lesions such as a subdural hematoma, or post-encephalitis, should be investigated, especially when the onset of the reading disability has been sudden.

In summary, there is ample evidence of the pathology involved with cerebral dysfunction, and there is also a suggestive relation between this dysfunction and learning disabilities: the CNS pathology and signs of learning disability and the signs of CNS dysfunction can be correlated. The characteristics that can be common to both conditions are (1) variability of performance, (2) concrete thinking but little abstract thinking, (3) perceptual motor impairment, (4) speech and language impairment, (5) motor awkwardness, (6) hyperkinesis and distractability, and (7) immaturity.

Aside from assisting in the drug therapy (see Chapter 5), which may be indicated in the treatment of some of these children for their hyperactivity, a pediatrician's goal should be to communicate and counsel with others who are working with the child. The pediatrician should act as a liaison between the family, the educator, and the psychologist. This may be the pediatrician's most important function with the child who has reading difficulty when the etiology is classified as brain damage or cerebral dysfunction.

REFERENCES

Birch, H., and Belmont, L. Auditory-visual integration in normal and retarded readers. *American Journal of Orthopsychiatry,* 1964, *34,* 852–861.

Dejerine, J. Contribution a l'etude anatamo-pathologique et clinique des differentes varies de cecite berbale. *Memoirs de la Société de Biologie,* 1892, *4,* 61.

Ford. F. *Diseases of nervous system in infancy.* Springfield, Illinois: Charles C. Thomas, 1966.

Gesell, A., and Amatruda, C. *Developmental diagnosis* (ed. 2). New York: Harper and Row, 1967.

Goldberg, H., Marshall, C., and Sims E. The role of brain damage in congenital dyslexia. *American Journal of Ophthalmology,* 1960, *50,* 486.

Hardy, J., and Peeples, M. Serum bilirubin levels in newborn infants: Distributions and associations with neurological abnormalities during the first year of life. *Johns Hopkins Medical Journal,* 1971, *128,* 265–72.

Kawi, A., and Pasamanik, B. Association of factors of pregnancy with the development of reading disorders in childhood. *Journal of the American Medical Association,* 1958, *166,* 1420.

Kennard, M., Rabinovitch, R., and Wexler, D. The abnormal electroencephalogram as related to reading disability in children with disorders of behavior. *Canadian Medical Association Journal,* 1952, *67,* 330–333.

Khoudadoust, A., Ziai, M., and Biggs, S. Optic disc in normal newborns. *American Journal of Ophthalmology,* 1968, *66,* 502–504.

Landau, L., and Benson, D. Cerebral palsy and mental retardation: Ocular findings. *Journal of Pediatric Ophthalmology,* 1971, *8,* 248.

Payne, R. Minimal chronic brain syndrome in children. *Developmental Medicine and Child Neurology,* 1962, *4:* 21.

Penfield, W., and Roberts, L. *Speech and brain mechanisms.* Princeton, New Jersey: Princeton University Press, 1959.

Prechtl, H., and Stemmer C. The choreiform ·syndrome in children. *Developmental Medicine and Child Neurology,* 1962, *4,* 119.

Rappaport, S. *Childhood aphasia and brain damage: Differential diagnosis* (Vol. 2). Narberth, Pennsylvania: Livingston Publishing Company, 1965.

Strauss, A., and Lehtinen, L. *Psychopathology and education of the brain injured child.* New York: Grune & Stratton, 1947.

Towbin, A. Organic causes of minimal brain dysfunction. *Journal of the American Medical Association,* 1971, *217,* 1207–1214.

Walsh, F., and Lindenberg, R. Hypoxia in children. *Bulletin of the Johns Hopkins Hospital,* 1961, *108,* 100–145.

5

Psychiatric Aspects

The question as to whether psychiatric disturbances can be a primary factor causing learning disabilities or whether the emotional disorders are a consequence of the child's learning disability needs to be considered.

Actually both situations are possible. Children faced with considerable emotional stress will not achieve to the level indicated by their learning potential. Similarly, the emotional problem can result from the children's inability to learn. In either case these children feel inadequate, frustrated, and guilty because of the lack of success in learning. Conflict and hostility between parents, teachers, and peers are frequent concomitants when children cannot achieve successfully.

The psychiatric factors that can lead to a learning disability usually result from (1) those factors arising during the preschool years and (2) those factors arising after entering school. The psychiatric factors experienced in the preschool period are compounded when the child enters shool and experiences the additional stresses of early education and the stresses that are associated with peer relationships and all of its complications. Among the factors to be dealt with in the preschool developmental period are (1) the child's physical condition, (2) motivation provided by the family, and (3) the socioeconomic background.

Five perinatal factors have been identified as stress producers: (1) low birth weight; (2) respiratory distress; (3) high serum bilirubin

59

level; (4) dysmaturity; and (5) anemic diatheses. The signs of these conditions are frequently present during the newborn period or the first year of life. In the preschool years the vulnerability to emotional stress of a child with a neurological problem accentuates educational problems.

The increase in emotional reactivity of individuals following brain injury is well accepted and Bender (1956), among others, has pointed out this emotional vulnerability of children with cerebral dysfunction. It has been shown that even a mild degree of brain damage can be the basis for behavioral disturbances manifested by a low frustration level, impulsiveness, and rapid mood swings.

Persistent illness, chronic infections, and other physical handicaps may create emotional stresses that may interfere with the child's reading readiness. Any difficulty in seeing or hearing will make reading more difficult and if not corrected in the preschool years will complicate and compound the problems of the emotionally disturbed child.

Traumatic events in the family environment can create emotional problems in children. The death of a parent, absence of a loved one, or divorce are difficult situations that are both immediate and lingering.

Such emotional trauma can also be true of a family situation that involves chronic alcoholism or a situation in which a parent has a continuing illness. There is no doubt that children fear for the health of a chronically ill parent and, if this anxiety continues into their school years, they may daydream and be out of contact with reality when the home situation competes for their attention. Their mind may wander to the home situation and they may tune out the classroom teacher.

Constant bickering within a family is equally traumatic to children. This is especially true if the children discover or think that they are unwanted and that they are the center of parental quarrels. When the child fails, the quarrels may become more bitter as one or the other of the parents is blamed for the failure. Furthermore, where the home situation is chaotic—for whatever reason—the children are often denied the emotionally stabilizing aspects of love, attention, and discipline that they need.

Many children from disadvantaged environments enter the public school system unprepared for the primary curriculum. This may be due to a variety of preschool factors including those of a social, economic, and cultural nature. Hess (1968) has found that "the initiative of the mother, and her tendency to meet the environment and to enter into interaction with it, appear to be important variables in the development of educability in the young child." The child from a culturally deprived lower economic environment may react negatively upon entering school if the environment and curriculum are predicated upon middle-class ideals. If the child is from a different ethnic group, his or her linguistic and cultural "differentness" may create even more emotional problems and frustrations.

After the child has started school, there are a number of other factors that produce emotional problems. Some are new factors and some relate to problems from the preschool years. The child who continues to be anemic or chronically ill cannot learn as well as he or she should. Where family difficulties (alcoholism, divorce problems, or family quarrels) continue into the school years, the child may daydream and "tune out" the teacher while his or her mind dwells upon the problems at home. When a child's ethnic, cultural, and socioeconomic background are different, the unfamiliarity with the school setting makes the child apprehensive and fearful because there are so many things which he or she cannot do or understand. If the child is physically immature or has been sheltered at home, his or her encounters with bullies and militant children in the school environment often create excruciating fears, resulting in inadequate learning.

Three other factors that often occur after the beginning of school are important contributors to psychiatric difficulties; (1) shifting to other school situations, (2) sibling rivalry, and (3) aggressive parents. These merit attention in some detail.

One of the problems with families who continuously move and with some contemporary busing programs lies in the inexplicable (to the small child) shift from a familiar to an unfamiliar environment. Changes in environment may place the child under emotional stress to adjust to new situations. All experiences, to some degree, create emotional stress. Adjusting to constantly moving or to being bussed from one place to another, having to accommodate to a new school environment, and having to adjust to new peer relationships and to chaotic conditions of bus rides and possibly longer travel time may all lead to problems. The traditional mobility of present day families also contributes to the anxieties of a child. A first grader or second grader who is forced to go from one state or region to another because of family, economic, or military transfer reasons, may have difficulty in adjusting to different teaching methods, differences in dialects, and differences in curriculum. Frequently, the child is uprooted in midyear. There may be difficulty in the family's settling down again, and the child who is enrolled in two or three schools in a year's time is at high risk of having difficulties.

Another major cause of consternation and failure in children is the factor of sibling rivalry. The fact that Mary has performed well in school does not mean that her younger brother John will do as well. Both teachers and parents often place extreme and unwarranted pressure upon the second child, when they are actually dealing with two individual children. One child may have a greater capacity for learning than the other, may learn at a faster rate, or be better motivated to learn. The sibling rivalry always sets up an unfair comparison and makes learning far more difficult for the younger child and occasionally for the older child, as well.

Related to this is the "aggressive parent situation." Not until a child is of school age does the parent see the child in real competition with other children. Until this age, the child has been in competition only at play, and there have been few standards of measure by which he or she could be compared. Perhaps another child did speak a little earlier or is a little more perceptive, but the parent can always rationalize an apparent inadequacy by saying, "Johnny walked earlier." Many times the parent never sees the whole picture, and it is not until the child enters school that established standards materialize against which the child can be compared with others of the same age. When this happens, the very desire of the parents to see their child excel may often lie at the heart of the child's inability to perform as well as other children. Such strong desire for achievement by the parents is usually accompanied by home tensions and anxieties that can readily affect the child's learning process.

When parents expect more than the child is capable of performing, trouble is in the offing. Such a child, unable to meet expectations, will exhibit emotional problems including resentment, hostility, and guilt. The child will carry a constant burden of guilt because he or she cannot measure up to the older brother or sister or to the parents' ideals. Often, with aggressive parents, the child is expected to perform at some ideal level merely to satisfy the parental ego. Such expectations may result in the child producing hostility and resentment toward a sibling or the parents themselves.

Spielberger (1966) divided students into two groups: high-anxiety students and low-anxiety students. He found that the failure in the high-anxiety group amounted to 20.2 percent, while the failure rate in the low-anxiety group was only 5.8 percent. Similar and more current studies using Spielberger's method provide support for the conclusion that apprehension and tension are factors in failure.

Certainly one should not constantly increase tensions by comparing a child with the sibling or parent who might have achieved a high measure of success in school. It is as unrealistic and damaging to demand performance beyond one's capabilities, and, because children are individuals, they should be evaluated as separate personalities. The overambitious and aggressive parent causes only confusion, apprehension, and failure in the child confronted by some ideal model or sibling rival.

The child who is beset with problems of this nature will react to his or her failures in a certain progression, or series of reactions, which may be summarized as follows: (1) a "couldn't care less" attitude, (2) a paranoid attitude toward his teacher, (3) marked feelings of inferiority, and, (4) a tendency toward emotional blocking and frank aggressiveness towards others.

If a child is failing and receiving no support, the child will normally reject the learning situation by possibly saying, "I just couldn't care less," "I just do not want to learn," or "It is not important." The child may also not verbalize any of these concerns but express them through actions of indifference and through rejection of the learning process.

If the matter of the child's failure is pursued by the parents or the teacher, the child may develop a paranoid reaction toward the teacher. The unresolved problem of failure is transferred to the teacher and the child then complains, "The teacher just picks on me," or "The teacher doesn't like me," or "I can't learn the way she teaches." Thus, for a number of reasons, teachers often become the focus of a child's failure.

When failure cannot be successfully transferred to the teacher, feelings of marked inferiority often follow. If the child continues to fail after the effort to blame the teacher has failed, the child may begin to accept the idea that he or she is at fault, especially after being told repeatedly that he or she is stupid and lazy and does not have the ability to perform satisfactorily. This may result in a loss of self-esteem and ego, and the subsequent step is emotional blocking and frank aggressiveness.

In this final stage, the child has to be forced to go to school. Once the child is in school he or she tunes out the teacher, daydreams, and tries to dismiss the tension and discomfort that results from this problem, thus emotionally blocking out any possible learning experience. If pressed to perform, the child reacts with undisguised hostility and aggressiveness, trying to destroy the learning situation that causes the emotional turmoil. At this point, the child may disrupt classes, bully other students, or smash classroom displays and furnishings. When these hostile and destructive tendencies are frustrated, the child plays "hooky," becomes a school dropout, and may become involved in delinquent behavior.

Whether the psychiatric problem is the cause of reading difficulty or a result of it, the introverted child may become more introverted, and the extroverted child may react in a belligerent manner that can end in serious problems of major delinquency. One critical result that is often manifested by both types is an utter dislike for reading, and the very sight of a book may cause the feeling of resentment. Breaking down these antagonisms requires parental cooperation.

Alarmed, puzzled, and defensive when their child does not do well in reading, some parents try to prove both to themselves and others that their child is not handicapped by setting out to teach or tutor the child. Understandably, the child is confused by this. He or she may be trying very hard to do the right thing, but simply does not have the tools. The result may be that the child begins to resent the parents. If the parents sit down again with him, even in a calm moment, the child no longer trusts them and fears an explosion is imminent. It has now become impossible for the parents to give any assistance at all.

The reading environment at home is most important, and an active cooperation between teacher, parent, and student is needed to help in these cases. But the teaching of reading is best left to professionals who are far less likely to become emotionally involved than is the parent.

The child who cannot read may appear in the pediatrician's office in a variety of symptomatic guises. Only rarely do the parents admit to the doctor that they are perplexed over their child's inability to read. Most commonly the chief complaint is disguised with reading difficulty mentioned only incidentally or not at all. The children who are intelligent are often able to disguise their inability to read by making use of auditory learning to memorize passages in reading assignments. As the nonreaders ascend through the primary grades, their problems multiply because most subject matter requires reading. It soon becomes impossible for them to solve arithmetic or social studies problems, simply because they cannot read the instructions, even though they may have the academic skills to solve the problems. The impression is one of general academic failure. They are likely to be considered mentally retarded or lazy.

Much has been said about the average student who is a poor reader in our school system; however, the child with a high intellectual capacity and who performs in an inadequate manner is also of considerable concern. This is the child who is in the bright or even gifted range but reads below grade level. This student may barely pass his or her subjects but may attend college because of an ability to compensate for his or her difficulty in reading but once there may have great difficulty, thus never reaching true potential. This tragic failure may be the result of an unrecognized reading disability and often accounts for the varying degrees of success or failure of college students who "just never found themselves." Success with therapy may be said to vary inversely with the length of time the problem has persisted. The child who has a major psychiatric problem will need psychiatric treatment concurrent with a remedial program, or may even need psychotherapy for an initial period in preparation of accepting help in reading.

The family is best advised to cease pressuring and to avoid home teaching, which usually proves frustrating to parents as well as to the child. They should concentrate on building a better relationship with the child by developing his or her self-confidence. At the same time, specific problems in family–child relations require understanding, an opportunity for expression, and sympathetic guidance from the physician or counselor.

There is reason to believe that methods for the early detection and habilitation of children with reading disorders may make a significant contribution to solving the problem of juvenile delinquency. The high rate of reading disability among delinquents suggests, at least, that some of their poor motivation and their antisocial behavior may be caused partly by the repeated frustration and failure which they experience from their reading difficulties.

It is also well recognized that males exceed females in reading disabilities by a frequency that varies from 3:1 to 10:1. The greater male incidence may be explained by the following possibilities:

1. Greater female maturity at the age of 6
2. Greater male incidence of central nervous system trauma
3. Greater motivation of females in the learning situation
4. Secondary emotional conflict in the male associated with the above three items

Having established that children do in fact react poorly to learning situations, because of factors that exist before and after beginning school, and after describing the ways in which children react to failure, it is important to establish some goals for their psychiatric care. These goals were best described by Kanner (1966) as the "Five R's" of psychotherapy: (1) relieve, (2) relate, (3) release, (4) relearn, and (5) relax.

Firstly, the family situation must be *relieved*. The home environment is basic and the emotional pressures there must be dealt with honestly and realistically. It is in this situation that a school counselor with an understanding of psychiatric factors as they relate to reading can be of extreme value in contributing to an understanding of the family situation. A visit to the home, a review of the child's work habits, a look at the contributions of father and mother to motivating the child, and the relationship of siblings to each other can do more to provide background material than many visits to the psychiatrist's office.

Whether the problem is alcohol, parental incompatibility, divorce, death, chronic illness, or simply sibling rivalry and overly ambitious parents, the family situation must be relieved. Both public and private agencies can be called in for help in some of these cases. Often, the family needs only reassurance that the child is not stupid, lazy, or brain damaged. An explanation of the reasonable expectancy level of performance is also important. Group conferences with the parents, even with the whole family, may be helpful in relieving the critical burden of emotional stress upon the child.

Secondly, one should *relate* to the child to let the child know that he or she has a friend. One should try to establish some rapport with the child to let the child feel that someone is sympathetically concerned about his or her problem. Above all, one should try to reinforce for the child those techniques and areas of learning in which he or she is proficient and through which he or she can expect some successes.

Thirdly, one should help the child to *release* his or her emotions. One should encourage the child to express how he or she feels about the learning situation, allowing the child to release emotions of frustration and resentment toward the teacher, parents, or fellow students. The child who has these feelings must be able to discuss them with someone; otherwise, the child will not have a good self-assessment or understanding of the difficulties.

Fourthly, one should help the child to learn his or her role in life and society, since the child should experience success and acceptance in his or her adopted life roles. Certainly there is evidence of talent and motivation in every child, which can be related to realistic goals of achievement and proficiency.

Finally, everyone should *relax*. With emotional tension eased, the child can approach learning problems better. Through better understanding of these problems, family and parental worries can be alleviated and more realistic expectations can be established that will help to better guide and instruct the child. The physician, the psychologist, the psychiatrist, and other professionals can act as relaxed go-betweens for all, so that everyone can feel that a common goal has been acquired to which the child can relate in a realistic way and progress satisfactorily. After all, the principle of any psychotherapy or, in a broader sense, of all mental hygiene is an effort to attempt to help a person to retain or regain optimal condition of comfort and smoothness of functioning. One cannot exist without the other: when there is no smoothness of functioning, there is no comfort; when there is no comfort, no smoothness or achievement can be expected.

REFERENCES

Bender, L. *Psychopathology of children with organic brain disorders.* Springfield, Illinois: Charles C. Thomas, 1956.

Blanchard, P. Psychogenic factors in some cases of reading disability. *American Journal of Orthopsychiatry,* 1935, *5,* 361–374.

Diethelm. O. and Jones, M. Influence of anxiety on attention, learning, retention and thinking. *Archives of Neurological Psychiatry,* 1947, *58,* 325–326.

Fabian, A. Clinical and experimental studies of school children who are retarded in reading. *Quarterly Journal of Child Behavior,* 1951, *3*:15.

Hess, R. D. *Maternal behavior and the development of reading readiness in urban Negro children.* Unpublished presentation at Claremont Reading Conference, Claremont, California, February 10, 1968.

Ingram, T., and Reid, I. Developmental aphasia observed in a department of child psychiatry. *Archives of the Disabled Child,* 1956, *31,* 161–172.

Kanner, L. *Child Psychiatry* (ed. 2). Springfield, Illinois: Charles C. Thomas, 1948.

Spielberger, D. *Anxiety and behavior.* New York: Academic Press, 1966.

6

The Role of Vision and Perception in Learning

Ophthalmologists who devote any part of their practice to the care of children will soon become aware that a great many patients in this group have various forms of reading disorders or are hyperactive, hyperkinetic, or have minimal brain dysfunction. They will also become aware of the fact that there is very little information in the ophthalmic literature about these various disorders. Often ophthalmologists are called upon to "do something" about the eyes because reading problems "obviously" must be related to the visual system. At other times, they will find themselves seeing a child who has been exposed to long periods of "eye exercises" that have been unsuccessful in remediating the child's learning problems.

The eye is one of the most adaptable structures of the body. An individual is not likely to injure the eyes simply by reading. One may read in glare or in diminished light or even watch television in a dark room for days on end, which may provoke fatigue and give evidence of eye strain but cannot injure eyesight. Let us take a brief look at the construction of the eye and the process of vision as it functions in the act of reading.

The eye consists of a transparent area called the cornea. Behind is the iris, which gives the eye its color. The dark pupil in the center of the iris is a circular space and is dark only because there is no light inside the vitreous cavity. Behind the iris is the lens, which is also transparent and shaped somewhat like a flattened sphere. It is suspended by a web of fine filaments and is capable of changing shape in order to focus on distant and near objects.

The center of the eyeball posterior to the lens is filled with vitreous humor, a fluid which is 99 percent water and makes up most of the eye's volume. This viscous jelly helps hold the eye's shape and keep the retina in place. The retina is a transparent tissue covering most of the inner aspects of the eye. When this covering is stimulated by light, it registers a chemical change. Light rays from any point outside the eye are bent by the interface as they pass from the air through the cornea. The rays are focused on the retina by the action of the lens and cornea. The retina consists of 6½ million cone cells that provide acute central vision and about 120 million rods that are color-blind but are more sensitive to light than the cones.

From the retina, electrochemical impulses convey the stimulus to the brain almost instantaneously. The frequency of the impulses informs us of the brilliance of light. Dim light causes less than 8 impulses per second in a nerve. Very bright light provokes 130 impulses per second in a nerve. Although the function of the eye can be compared with a camera, the retina is not like a photographic plate in that it registers only a temporary chemical change, which disappears in about one tenth of a second.

If everything that has been mentioned to this point functions properly, one still could not read unless the eyes could move constantly and quickly, every tenth of a second. Eye movement is controlled by a set of six muscles. The eyes constantly sweep across the object of focus and interest with micronystagmoid fixations. Since the image on the retina lasts for only about one tenth of a second, we do not notice the jerkiness. The eyes move in tandem to see objects, like the front wheels of a car. Sharp images of objects must be formed no matter what the distance from the eye. For this purpose the lens is pliable and often changes its shape. This ability is known as accommodation, and the extent to which the eye can perform this task is defined as accommodative power or amplitude of accommodation.

But beyond the mechanical functioning of the eye, the process of seeing is not complete until what is seen is interpreted by the observer. This is called perception and is an interpretation that is based on past experience. This is entirely a function of the brain.

Far too much emphasis is generally placed on the importance of good vision as it affects children who have reading problems. There is no definite evidence of any relationship between visual ability and reading problems. Yet, nearly every classroom teacher (as well as many reading specialists) would like to think that when a child has a problem in reading, the correction of a visual defect, whether by the use of glasses or by the use of muscle exercises, will be a substantial aid to solving the reading problem. In fact, many highly regarded reading specialists have been misled to the extent that they have suggested the use of eye exercises as a helpful aid in reading problems.

A visual defect does not mean that the visual inefficiency is causing the reading problem. Some students with extremely poor vision are excellent readers. There is no conclusive evidence as to the connection of any eye disorder with the ability to read, or even with scholastic achievement in other areas. It is appropriate that schools give visual screening tests to detect visual disorders and make the condition known to parents, since they may contribute to "slow reading" due to an inability to identify quickly the written symbol.

There are a number of screening tests used by schools for detection of visual defects. The most frequently used is the Snellen chart, which measures visual acuity or sharpness of vision. The test determines the smallest letter that can be read at a distance of 20 feet. A visual acuity of 20/20 which is considered normal, simply means that at 20 feet the observer can read a letter 8.86 millimeters square. An acuity score of 20/30 means that at 20 feet the smallest letter the observer can read is one that should have been seen normally at 30 feet.

Another test used is the Keystone Visual Survey (Keystone View Company, Davenport, Iowa) and the Titmus Tester (Titmus Optical Company, Petersburg, Virginia) which goes further in testing depth perception and muscle balance. Such tests show whether the eyes are working together. Some schools use a Binocular Reading Test, which reveals the extent to which each eye sees print when both eyes are in use.

Still another test is made possible by the ophthalmograph. This device uses a camera to photograph the simultaneous movements of both eyes. A careful interpretation of the film reveals certain patterns as indications of reading habits. The graph will clearly demonstrate if one eye wanders from the print or if the eyes may have to make adjustments to find the beginning of a line of print. It demonstrates the number of fixations a child must make in order to read a line of printed material.

When a child's vision is impaired, it is important that the condition receive competent diagnosis and treatment because a child with poor sight will have difficulty identifying details of the printed page. In the case of poor visual acuity, the condition could be corrected by the use of glasses.

Refractive visual defects most often include far-sightedness (hyperopia) and near-sightedness (myopia). Normal eyes can see an image 20 feet or more away clearly when the ciliary muscles of the eyes used for focusing are relaxed. The far-sighted person has a near point of clear vision that is farther away than the person with normal vision. He or she cannot see a near object clearly without accommodating to focus on the object. The near-sighted person can see clearly at only a short distance when the focusing muscles are relaxed. This distance may vary from a few feet to as short a distance as a few inches. Both conditions can be corrected with lenses. The defect known as astigmatism is one that causes objects to appear distorted. This can be caused by a defect in the curvature of the cornea or lens. This condition also can usually be corrected with lenses.

The most common of the muscle disorders of the eye is the condition known as strabismus. With this condition there may be a horizontal deviation, as when one eye is turned in or one eye is turned out, or a vertical deviation when one eye is turned up or down. The unused eye, as a result of suppression, may suffer from varying degrees of visual impairment. This may result in a condition called amblyopia ex anopsia, or poor vision as a result of cortical suppression. Glasses help in many cases—but not in all. Other cases can be helped with surgery, during which the deviating eye is moved to the correct position.

OCULAR MOTILITY

There are four systems concerned with ocular motility. They have to do with the saccadic, pursuit, vergence, and vestibular. A word of description is necessary since these symptoms are frequently discussed when a child has a learning disability.

Saccadic movement describes a rapid movement of the eye

when one sees a peripheral stimulus and an effort is made to bring the object or word into focus on the macula. The movement is provided by a burst of energy of the agonist muscles and a complete inhibition of the antagonist muscle. The nerve stimulus emerges from the frontal lobes of the brain. The right frontal lobe is responsible for horizontal conjugate gaze to the left and conversely, the left frontal lobe is responsible for horizontal gaze to the right. Both frontal lobes are active in vertical saccades; therefore, no defect of vertical saccades are seen in unilateral hemispheric lesions. The pathway of the nerve fiber tracts are by way of the frontomesencephalic pathway. The horizontal saccades course from the frontal lobe to the opposite paramedian pontine reticular formation crossing at the level of the oculomotor nuclei.

The vertical saccades have their innervation from both frontal lobes to the pretectal area. The characteristics of the saccadic movement are:

1. Rapid eye movements
2. Long delay from stimulus to execution
3. Preprogrammed movement
4. Movement that is usually precise but a slight undershoot or overshoot is normal
5. Electromyograms that show an abrupt increase in activity of agonist, and an immediate silence of the antagonist
6. Movement that is moderated by the cerebellum

If there is a cerebellar lesion there is a loss of precision of saccadic movements; in other words, ocular dysmetria, ocular flutter, and opsoclonus.

The pursuit system is slow and is concerned with maintaining fixation. It is represented in the occipito-parietal lobe. The right occipital lobe is responsible for motion to the left. The pathway is from the occipital lobe to the brain stem reticular formation crossing mostly at the level of the third and fourth nuclei terminating in the pontine gaze center.

The characteristics of pursuit movements are:

1. Slow movement
2. Short delay from stimulus to execution
3. Continuous monitoring system
4. **EMG demonstrates increasing contraction of the agonist and gradual relaxation of the antagonist**

Pursuit movement is responsible for following or tracking a slowly and smoothly moving target once the saccadic movement places it on the fovea.

Lesions in the central nervous system will cause interruption of smooth movement with replacement by saccades. The vergences have to do with nonparallel movement. The cortical representation is in the occipito-parietal area and is characterized by very slow nonparallel or disconjugate movements. Additionally, the function of the vestibular system is to coordinate eye and head movements while OKN or opticokinetic nystagmus is an ocular phenomenon produced by repeated pursuit movements.

All of these movements can be summarized in the following story. A duck hunter went hunting with a very astute ophthalmologist who made the following observations: While the men were sitting in the duck blind, there was a sudden sound and their eyes made a "saccadic" rapid motion to get a fix on the flying ducks. Then the hunter followed the flying targets with a "pursuit" movement. In order to aim his rifle there was a "vergence" motion as he converged on the rifle sight. Then as he shot, the boat began to rock and he used his "vestibular" system to coordinate the eye and head movements. As the ducks flew away, "opticokinetic nystagmus" was produced by repeated fixations on the flying ducks.

Schools are often pressured by consultants, parents, and influential board members to adopt one or another approach as an aid in teaching reading. Since many of the recommendations for treatment of learning disabilities include "eye exercises," it is important that professionals investigate some of the techniques which have been prescribed and are being used by some disciplines.

VISION

Some members of the optometric profession have continually emphasized that vision consists of vision plus perception. It is well known that vision consists of the peripheral aspects, which include acuity, muscle balance, fusion, and near point convergence. The central aspects of vision involve the organizing of the visual stimuli until conception and understanding occurs.

It is advantageous and appropriate to interpret tactile, auditory, olfactory, gustatory and other appropriate proprioceptive experiences with the visual experience. Each of these proprioceptive impulses do in fact reinforce each other and the learning experience. It is questionable to speak of visual development occurring only through movement. There are numerous examples of children in a clinical setting who although restricted in movement acquire the ability to read quite proficiently. The statement that movement is necessary for visual development is questionable. There is no question that the act of writing the word "boy" can be enhanced and memorized more easily if kinesthetic and tactile stimuli are used for reinforcement. This is not to say that the word could not be learned without reinforcement by proprioceptive stimuli.

Gross and fine motor control reflect the organization of the central nervous system. The feedback of somesthetic cues from muscles and joints contribute to the sense of body position. Optimal gross motor control enhances self-esteem but there is little evidence of a direct relationship between effective motor function and early learning of basic academic skills. Lack of fine motor performance, however, may affect the ability to write, copy from the blackboard, and grasp a pencil.

The ophthalmograph and later the electronystagmograph were developed to record ocular movements during reading. The characteristics of the reading habit and the nature of binocular motor coordination during reading could be interpreted from a reading graph. While the technique was good, the analysis of the resulting graphs suffered from misinterpretation: it was claimed that the faulty eye movements represented on these graphs were the cause of poor reading.

Routine muscle tests were thought to be inferior to the ophthalmographic record because in the former the eye movements were not measured in the actual reading situation. It was thought that the muscle test created a special visual situation under which the eyes were then measured. The objection was that these relationships were interpreted in terms of a wider functional ability than the scope of the test would allow.

The relative importance of good ocular movement to good reading becomes apparent when it was claimed that the smoother and more accurate the binocular activity, the faster and more efficient was the reading. Inadequate understanding of this relationship and of the implications of the reading graph may result in educators suggesting orthoptic or muscle exercises in an effort to train ocular movement, believing that this would be beneficial in improving reading. A common practice is to obtain the child's reading graph in the first grade, expose him or her to the tachisto-scope or perhaps some form of exercise, and then retest the child's ocular movements at the end of the academic session. It is claimed that improvement in ocular motility is the reason for the child's improved reading ability.

In 1950, the American Optical Company Bureau of Visual Science claimed that various abnormalities indicated on a series of graphs were the cause of certain cases of reading failure. Lengthy fixations indicated slow reaction to the printed material. It was claimed that exercise with the tachistoscope resulted in better control of eye movements and improved reading ability. Abnor-malities of excessive convergence, it was said, resulted in a lack of rhythm in the reading pattern and a consequently poor reading ability.

To investigate this subject, the present authors examined the eye movements of 50 reading disabled children and a matched number of normal children to serve as controls. The apparatus used for the study was the electronystagmograph, a machine which measures the difference in the electrical potential between the retina and cornea synchronous with ocular movements. Each child was asked to read material below his or her frustration level, and a graph was obtained. Then the child was asked to read material above his frustration reading level (see Figure 6-1). The obtained graph demonstrated abnormalities that varied with the difficulty of the word or sentence and resulted in changes on the graph which were synchronous with difficulties in the reading material (see Figure 6-2).

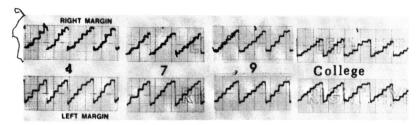

Figure 6-1. Normal Reader. Demonstration of normal myograph at fourth, seventh, ninth, and twelfth year reading levels.

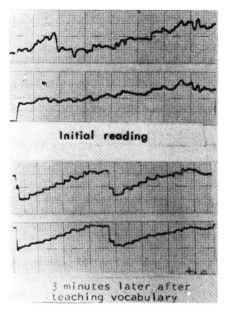

Figure 6-2.   Disabled Reader. Myograph tracings demonstrating poor reading ability (two upper tracings) and subsequent improvement in ability three minutes after vocabulary was taught.

Two additional parts of the experiment were designed. Shadow reading—reading with the child—was done and graphs obtained as the child read both below frustration and above frustration material. In all cases, the ocular movements became symmetrical and improved toward the normal pattern.

In another study, frustration words were taught in advance of reading the material. Within minutes after this previously frustrating material was read, the graph showed definite improvement over previous untutored graph recordings. In actuality, it is not the eyes that read, but it is the brain that reads (see Figures 6-3 and 6-4).

In summary, the electronystagmograph and the ophthalmograph provide convenient methods for analyzing ocular movements. Findings indicate that it is the degree of comprehension that produces the type of ocular movement, not ocular motility that determines the degree of comprehension. When the child had difficulty in understanding the word or the syllable, he or she would

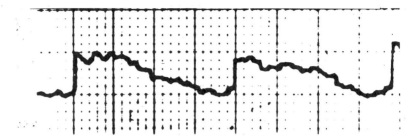

Figure 6-3. Japanese physician reading Japanese language material. Note normal myograph pattern.

exhibit regression of eye movement or often a prolonged fixation as he attempted to reconstruct the word. As soon as the child was able to understand the words, reading resumed in normal fashion. This evidence suggests that it is the ability to understand that determines the fluidity of the reading and that ocular motility simply denotes the degree of fluidity. The electronystagmograph provides a method of studying these ocular movements. It is important to note that this research was done under monocular and binocular conditions, using the electronystagmograph. Improving ocular motility has become a widely discussed technique of assisting children who have learning disabilities. It has been assumed that learning difficulties, in some

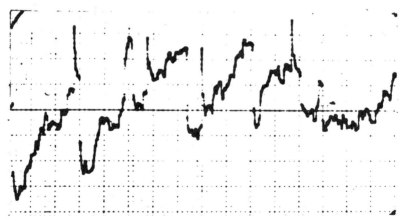

Figure 6-4. Japanese physician reading third grade level English. Note the irregularities in the waveform.

cases, were due to lack of binocular coordination. While the electronystagmograph and ophthalmograph do demonstrate incoordinate eye movements in children who have difficulty in reading, the experiments performed demonstrate that improper eye movements seem to be the result rather than the cause of poor comprehension.

An interesting example of eye movements concerns the inability of people who are blind from birth to move their eyes in any direction. Additionally, people who are blind from birth have no visual dreams. If, however, they are blinded after adolescence, they can move their eyes perfectly normally in all directions even though they are blind. When they attempt to follow a finger, they will have normal pursuit movements and will have dreams that include the visual system. The conclusions that can be drawn from this example are that ocular movements are controlled by the brain and certainly not controlled by the eyes.

Ocular patching, or filtration, has become a very much discussed method of stimulating learning in those children who might have crossed dominance. The following discussion will attempt to demonstrate the fallacy of such methods.

Inhibition plays a necessary and vital part in integrating a final perceptual pattern. If two similar images are presented to corresponding retinal points in each eye, the images are fused, and the final perceptual pattern is a fused single image. If the images are grossly dissimilar and are presented to corresponding points on the retina so that they cannot be fused into one perceptual pattern, one of the images is suppressed and is eliminated from consciousness. When the images are of equal stimulus, a condition of retinal rivalry exists.

If the two eyes are equal, inhibition of one macula occurs when the other occupies the focus of interest. A state of rivalry results, and the inhibition is temporary and conditioned only by use of the other eye. This occurs only during binocular activity. Either eye may function, alternately retaining good vision when in use and reverting to perceptual blindness when the other eye does the seeing. The site of the suppression seems to be the result of a cortical inhibition.

Binocular fixation of two retinal images is the act of maintaining these images on corresponding retinal points by means of motor responses to these images (fusion movements). The most elementary type of binocularity (simultaneous perception) occurs when the two images, as seen by the two eyes, are superimposed to form one image. In the second grade of binocularity there is true fusion with some amplitude, and here not only are the two images fused, but some effort is made to maintain this fusion in spite of difficulties. In the third grade (or highest type) of binocularity the images of the two eyes are fused and blended to produce a stereoscopic effect. This is on the perceptual level.

Patching, or filtration, is a technique in which red and green filters are used in conjunction with red and green printed material. If the green glass is over the right eye and the red glass over the left eye, the red and green material which is on the page will alternately be neutralized and, therefore, will not be seen. Thus, we can stimulate either one eye or the other. The theory is that if the child is right-handed, right-footed, and left-eyed, an attempt is made to convert the controlling or dominant left eye to the right side, to correspond with the right-handedness and right-footedness.

There is no evidence that crossed dominance impedes learning. Both hemispheres receive visual stimuli from both eyes, and ocular dominance does not indicate that only one hemisphere is functioning. All impulses that come in by way of the right eye are actually perceived with both sides of the brain. Similarly, all impulses that come in by way of the left eye are also seen by both sides of the brain. This occurs because there is a decussation or crossing of the optic nerve fibers in the optic chiasm. When we see with either the right or left eye, both sides of the brain are receiving sensations. If there is damage to one hemisphere, the patient will develop a hemianopsia or half visual field. This is not true in dyslexia or with any children who have reading problems.

The question should be asked, what happens to the impulse after it arrives at the occipital cortex? To demonstrate this, a simple experiment in retinal rivalry can be performed. A red glass is placed over the right eye and a green glass over the left eye. When a target is fixated, there is rapid red and green alteration of stimulus as the impulse is received, first by the right eye and then by the left eye. This same phenomenon can be represented by means of a machine called the amblyoscope. If a stimulus, such as a lollipop, is first presented to one eye, and then another image, such as the mouth of the child, is presented to the opposite eye, the first degree of binocular fusion would present itself as being the lollipop in the mouth of the child. The frequency with which either stimulus is seen has nothing to do with dominance or the rate of learning.

The philosophy of muscle exercises lies in the expectation that the eyes can coordinate better and the patient can be taught better visual and perceptive habits, and thus be enabled to read better. The exercises start with teaching one eye to move freely, then teaching the other eye to move freely. After this freedom of monocular vision has been established, the same process is attempted with both eyes working together. The attempt is then made to improve the facility of accommodative change, that is, to develop the ability to focus freely from far to near and back again. The procedure is called "accommodative rock." These exercises also attempt to establish stereopsis, or depth perception, for both far and near objects. They attempt to eliminate suppressions of either eye, to build fusion reserves, and establish hand-eye coordination. In addition to being expensive, it is now becoming clear that eye exercises have no supportive data to suggest they aid the reading disabled child. The only benefit one might receive is the increased motivation that will come from the attention and understanding he gets during the "reading therapy."

In conclusion, parents and teachers are urged to remember how tough and adaptable the human eye is. It is impossible to injure the eye by reading or looking in any way. On the other hand, if there is an ocular defect, it should be corrected, but eye exercises will not improve one's ability to read. Eyes receive a peripheral sensory stimulus, and any normal pair of eyes does that job easily, continuously, and without conscious upkeep or care. We can assume that lack of normal vision (within limits, of course, people cannot read what they cannot see) is not a cause of reading problems. Poor vision may make children slow readers because they have difficulty identifying details, but it will not produce reversals or make them delayed readers. Correction of the visual problem may increase speed of reading, but it will not increase perceptive abilities.

Optometric thought on this subject seems to be divided into two groups. Most optometrists confine their role in educational achievement to visual enhancement for the sake of clear, comfortable, and efficient visual performance. Some follow the "developmental vision" point of view, feeling that learning in general and reading in particular are primarily visual-perceptual tasks. This group advocates "visual training" in cases of reading disability.

VISUAL TRAINING

"Visual training" is often defined in terms of perceptual training even though therapy is directed toward peripheral training. Some
of the peripheral visual abilities that are claimed to be trainable are
(1) the ability to follow smoothly and accurately with both eyes; (2)
the ability to fixate quickly and accurately with both eyes on a series
of fixed objects; (3) the ability to change focus quickly and without
blur from far to near and from near to far; and (4) the ability to
maintain attention for extended periods of time at near-point activity. In the more technical language of ocular dynamics, these
abilities are classified as fixation ability, fusion, stereopsis, binocularity, and motility patterns.

There is the possibility that some children improve in reading
ability when visual training and tutoring are combined. Adequately
controlled studies that would indicate that visual training alone is
correlated with an increase of reading ability are lacking.

THE PERCEPTUAL ASPECTS OF VISION

When a child has a reading disability, his or her eyes are
immediately considered as a possible cause of the difficulty. Since a
visual defect might contribute to slower learning, it should be
corrected because such treatment makes reading more comfortable
for the child. There is now, however, general agreement that factors
of visual acuity, refractive error, eye muscle imbalance, binocularity, or fusion are only peripheral and are not causative factors in
reading disability. In comparisons between groups of normal readers
and disabled readers, no peripheral visual factors has been found to
have a higher incidence in one group than in the other. In fact,
investigations have proven that peripheral visual factors are irrele-
vant to the basic problem of reading disability and should not be
considered as causes of a child's learning difficulty. Consequently,
in the past few years, many educators and others interested in the
field of learning have turned their attention from the eye and
peripheral ocular functions as a cause of failures to the broader area
of visual perception.

Anatomically, perception is the sum of what takes place from
the time a visual impression is received peripherally by the eye until

it is transmitted to, recorded by, and understood in the brain. This same type of stimulation is also transmitted into the brain from the areas of hearing, touch, smell, and joint positional sense. It is in the brain that all of these impulses are received, decoded, and organized so that perception and cognition take place. Because visual perception is so important in the learning and reading processes, visual perception deserves further attention (Norn et al., 1969).

Expressed one way, visual perception is the ability to recognize and discriminate visual stimuli and to interpret them correctly in the light of previous experiences. In another sense, visual perception is a process whereby peripheral sensory stimuli are organized in the brain. Visual perception then is not the ability to see accurately, but is the interpretation of what is "seen" by the brain. For example, if one looks at the four lines that form a square, a sensory impression is received on the retina of each eye. The impulses are transmitted from the retina and are recorded in the occipital lobe of the brain. These are the peripheral visual factors that are sensory to the brain, but it is the function of the brain to recognize and classify these lines as a "square," a significant geometric form.

To use a different illustration, visual perception is a process that begins when the peripheral factors have been recorded in the occipital lobe and then transmitted to the angular gyrus of the parietal lobe. Here, an animal is perceived as a four-legged beast, and once this has happened, it is possible to differentiate among four-legged beasts. It is not until the information goes through the parietal lobe to the frontal lobe of the brain that a cow or a horse can be differentiated through an understanding of their functions. This is conception or understanding. Thus, it is the brain that must provide an accurate conception and understanding of what is seen.

A child may see the words "horse" and "house" on the printed page, but it is through a very complex process that the visual impression is translated and organized in the brain. Perception becomes meaningful when the child recognizes the difference in these words. Reading with understanding can take place when the child has the ability to recognize differences in words and can comprehend and understand their different meanings.

There are certain abilities that a child develops in a definite sequence, normally at certain age levels. First, there is the sensory-motor phase. This comprises the initial 18 months and constitutes that period of life when a child first becomes aware of the world around him or her, through movement combined with the use of all of the senses. The second phase is the language phase, which often begins in the second year of life. It is characterized by a rapid development of speech. Here the child learns to develop and to express ideas through speech. This is the point of the child's development where there is most apt to occur some deficit in the visual and auditory sequencing.

Following this phase of maximum language development, the maximum development of perceptual ability occurs. The perceptual phase spans the period from 3 to about 6 years of age. Piaget (1952) refers to perception as the intuitive aspects of intelligence as perception enables a child to recognize objects around him or her, directly and intuitively, without deliberation and without simultaneous use of movement. Among the abilities developing during this period are those perceptual skills necessary for discriminating two-dimensional figures. The fourth phase in the child's development, the phase of concrete operation, begins when the child is about 6 years of age. At this point the child begins to associate his or her present experiences with his or her previous knowledge.

Visual-perceptual skills usually develop from birth to the age of 6 in a sequential pattern (Piaget, 1952). If a child does not develop the perceptual skills before the age of 6, he or she may be at risk for learning difficulties. It is important to know this and to be able to test children during this developmental period. For example, if a child sees a "b" as a "d" or "24" as "42" or if from an auditory point of view, a child hears the correct sound but if in transferring this sensory impression the brain receives a faulty impression, then the child is in difficulty. The child's interpretation of letters and symbols is distorted, and therefore his or her ability to read and correctly interpret what he or she reads is impaired. It is possible that this child has a lag in the development of perceptual skills.

There are many methods of examining visual-perception ability. The Bender-Motor Gestalt Test, originated by Lauretta Bender, and adapted for use with children, as described by Koppitz (1963), has been one of the primary methods of investigation in the visual-perceptual area. In the language development phase, many diagnosticians still use the Illinois Test of Psycholinguistic Abilities (ITPA). A principle test for evaluation of a child's higher cognitive functions is usually the Wechsler Intelligence Scale for Children-Revised (WISC-R).

Another frequently used instrument for examining visual perception in children was developed by Marianne Frostig, known as the Frostig Perceptual Tests. These tests involve evaluations in: eye-motor coordination, figure-ground perception, constancy of visual perception, perception of position in space, and perception of space relationships.

EVALUATING PERCEPTUAL FACTORS IN READING DISABILITY

A study by Goldberg (1972) found that visual sequential memory was significantly correlated with several measures of reading. Some of these correlations were found to be positive and significant, even after the effects of chronological age were removed from the correlations. The intercorrelations suggest that a reading disability may result from a lack of coordination among the three different visual functions required for reading: visual memory, visual sequencing, and visual perception.

The child of 6 years or older, whose perceptual-motor, visual-motor, and conceptual performance is relatively primitive, is the one who is likely to run into difficulty when exposed to reading. Based on this line of reasoning, "copying" tests may be useful as part of a battery when screening for reading readiness, predicting school achievement, and diagnosing reading and learning problems.

The ophthalmologist or pediatrician engaged in routine practice is not qualified to do highly specialized educational testing. Additionally, tests such as the Bender-Gestalt and the Frostig Test should be administered by trained specialists. It has become important, however, for ophthalmologists and pediatricians to understand educational tests as they increasingly hear about them in routine practice.

It has been well documented that perceptual training after the age of 6 years is of questionable value in the treatment of learning disorders (Bettman et al., 1967). Time spent in the teaching of reading might accomplish greater benefits than time spent in perceptual training. Such training could be of benefit at the ages of 1 to 6 years in the reading readiness stage, but after this period the child makes his or her own compensations to residual deficits.

Perceptual training is analogous to a condition called amblyopia exanopsia. In this condition, a child does not develop normal visual acuity of one eye. It is accurate to say that there is no ocular pathology but that poor vision is due to a central cortical suppression of the visual image of one eye. If this condition is diagnosed before the child is 6 years of age, proper treatment will restore the vision to normal. If it is not diagnosed and treated before this age, then amblyopia (poor vision) most often is permanent. Similarly, if a child has a perceptual deficiency that is not diagnosed and treated before the age of 6, then perceptual training will probably not develop the skill that is lacking. The child may learn to read but the perceptual deficit may persist even if reading ability increases (Silver and Hagin, 1967).

REFERENCES

Bender, L. The Bender visual-motor gestalt test for children. Los Angeles: Western Psychological Services, 1962.

Bettman, J., Stein, E., Whitsell, L. & Gofman, H. Cerebral dominance in developmental dsylexia: The role of ophthalmology. *Archives of Ophthalmology,* 1967, *78,* 722–730.

Fernald, G. *Remedial techniques in basic school subjects.* New York: McGraw-Hill, 1943.

Frostig, M. *Frosting developmental test of visual perception.* Palo Alto, CA: Consulting Psychologists Press, 1963.

Frostic, M., Lefeuer, M., & Whattlesey, J. The Marianne Frostig developmental test of visual perception. Palo Alto, CA: Consulting Psychologists Press, 1964.

Goldberg, H., and Schiffman, G. *Dyslexia.* New York: Grune & Stratton, Inc. 1972.

Koppitz, E. *The Bender-Gestalt test for young children.* New York: Grune & Stratton, Inc., 1963.

Norm, M., Rindzinsky, E., & Skydsgaard, H. Ophthalmologic and orthoptic examinations of dyslectics. *Acta Ophthalmologica,* 1969, *47,* 147.

Piaget, J. *The origins of intelligence.* New York: International Universities Press, 1952.

Silver, A., and Hagin, R. Strategies of intervention in the spectrum of defects in specific reading disability. *Bulletin of the Orton Society,* 1967.

7

The Role of Dominance

In general animals are nearly always ambidextrous and show no preference for a particular paw or foot. The human species was originally ambidextrous as well. A study of cave paintings and tools employed by stone age man has revealed that there were about as many right-handed as left-handed individuals among our remote ancestors.

Right-dominance suddenly appeared in the Bronze Age. The reason for this is unknown, but there is a "weapon theory," which speculates that the right-handed individuals of the hunter-warrior stone age period survived because they carried their weapons in the right hand and protected their hearts by means of a shield. In any event, we know that the priority of the right hand was established in man during the Bronze Age because their scythes were designed for wielding by right-handed individuals.

The emergence of laterality in mankind, with dominance of one side of the body, usually the right eye, right hand and right foot, under the control of the left cerebral hemisphere, is a subject that has been fully explored and has had numerous social interpretations. In discussing facial asymmetry, for example, it has been suggested that the right half of the face is imprinted with the individual's attitudes toward life, while the left half expresses those traits of temperament that are governed by the individual's subconscious processing. It has been said that each of us is divided into a "left person,'' which is more light-hearted and more extroverted, and a "right person," which is more introverted and meditative.

Texts taken from the *Bible* and from the *Iliad* show that the distinction between right-handed and left-handed men has aroused the curiosity of researchers from earliest times. It is important to state that right/handed and left/handed persons are not simply mirror images of each other. Most persons are right-handed individuals whose language centers are situated in the left hemisphere of the brain. Dominance of the right foot is usually associated with dominance of the right hand. Left-handed persons, however, may have language centers located in the right hemisphere of the brain.

Many investigators (Geschwind, 1972; Wada, 1969) have described in detail the successive stages through which the growing child passes before the right-handed or left-handed tendency becomes permanently established. The precise age of handedness is subject to great individual variation.

Handedness and language develop earlier in girls than in boys. This is to be expected because of the greater maturity of females at this stage of development. One can conclude that, generally, hand differentiation begins in the child at about nine months and may be complete by two years of age.

Dominance of the left hand occurs in approximately five to ten percent of the population of the United States. Left-hand dominance is twice as common in boys than in girls, and it is twice again as common in the retarded. Left-handedness is frequently associated with perinatal distress and also with abnormal EEG findings.

Handedness results not only from a possible genetic source, but also from the relationship of this handedness inheritance to parental attitudes. These parental attitudes toward handedness result from the social, vocational, economic, and educational experiences of the parents. Pure left-handedness is extremely rare. In a study by Subirana (1961), only one case out of 316 was found. The fact is that pure right-handedness is also rare. In this same group of 316 children, only 25 cases of pure right-handedness were found.

Right-handed individuals tend to write from left to right, while some left-handed persons tend to mirror-write from right to left. The Phoenicians wrote from right to left, as did their Semitic successors. The Greeks often had to reverse the orientation of their left-to-right script. This actually produced a period of writing lines in alternate directions, called Boustrophedon, which is after the pattern of ox plowing. By the fourth century B.C., however, both Greek and Roman writings were uniformly right-handed (dextrad).

The relationship between "handedness" and "eyedness" is very interesting. Man is primarily and innately right-eyed or left-eyed and only secondarily right- or left-handed. Ninety percent of individuals are right-handed but only two thirds of them are both right-handed and right-eyed. Left-eyedness occurs in 30 percent of individuals.

Most individuals have a preference for monocular sighting and this preference is established earlier than hand preference. The master eye is usually the one with better visual acuity. In some persons, the optically weaker eye may be preferred for sighting. In dominance, eyedness is a more significant finding because the person is not aware of his or her preferred eye and environmentally is not encouraged to change this dominance.

Artists are usually right-handed and, when painting in the daylight, they tend to position the window on their left side. The model is placed somewhat to the painter's left and nearer to the window, which illuminates the right side of the model's face. The model's right eye, or the master eye, looks directly at the artist and the left eye is allowed the freedom of a little divergence. When an artist paints a self-portrait, the right side of the face is illuminated but the left eye appears to be the master eye.

Dominance of the right eye was first noted in 1883 by Lombroso. This eye preference probably underlies foot and hand dominance, since the eye controls the hand. All three, the foot, the hand, and the eye, are related to the opposite side of the cerebral hemisphere. There is no absolute separation of left and right, and many interweaving grades of ambidexterity exist. The laterality of the brain is something that is genetically induced, generally as a recessive trait.

Another aspect of cerebral dominance is the dominance of the field of vision that corresponds to the master eye. There is a greater ease in directional scanning toward that field of vision. Persons with right-hand dominance find the right-hand side of the page easier to register, and the eyes sweep more easily to that side than away from it.

The concept of hemispheric cerebral localization is found in the Hippocratic writings of 400 B.C., which made the observation that a wound in the left temple produces a spasm in the opposite side of the body. The French researcher Pourfour du Petit demonstrated this fact experimentally in animals in 1710, and Morgagni, the great Italian anatomist, established it for man in the same century.

The concept of cerebral hemispheric dominance has emerged within the last 100 years or so. It arose out of Broca's observation in 1861 of the association between aphasia and lesions of the left frontal lobe. Broca's observations were made with extreme caution, and it was not until 1865 that Broca finally advanced the idea that aphasia was specifically related to disease of the left hemisphere.

At this time Broca postulated a relationship between handedness and hemispheric cerebral dominance for language. There was some question as to what the role of minor, or nondominant, hemisphere might be. There were some who thought that it might be a silent partner, participating in a supportive way in normal speech and capable of assuming the other function of speech mediation if the dominant hemisphere was out of action due to injury or disease. Others felt that the lesser hemisphere was the center for musical language. Still others have felt that the lesser cerebral hemisphere embraces a much broader range of activity.

The two hemispheres of the brain are joined anatomically together at several points. One is at the common stem that descends from the brain into the spinal cord, otherwise known as the medulla oblongata. Two other areas of possible junction are at the optic chiasm and at the cerebellum. A fourth connection, known as the great cerebral commissure, is made by means of the corpus collosum, and in this area much experimentation is taking place.

A task is learned in one of two ways: (1) by one hemisphere transmitting the information to the other at the time the initial learning takes place, or (2) by supplying it on demand later. In the first instance, intercommunication by way of the corpus collosum at the time of the learning results in the formation of a double set of memory traces, one in each half of the brain. In the second case, a set of engrams is established only in the directly trained half, but this information is available to the other hemisphere, when it is required, by way of the corpus collosum.

It was thought at one time that the corpus collosum was crucial for the proper performance of brain functions. It has been noted recently, however, that the corpus collosum can be cut in humans and in animals without any loss of function. In fact, the two halves of the brain can learn diametrically opposite solutions to the same experimental problem.

Sectioning of the corpus collosum, a procedure that prevents communication between the two halves of the brain, could demonstrate the interaction between the two hemispheres. If a normal animal is trained to do a trick with one paw, it can be shown that he will also know this trick with the left paw, and even a sectioning of the corpus collosum will not prevent its being known by the right paw. If, however, the section is made before the trick is learned by one paw, it has to be learned all over again by the other.

Proof of the fact that animal experiments in memory do not apply absolutely to man is suggested by the evidence that patients who are operated on for intractable epilepsy, by cutting the commissures, will have their epilepsy cured but suffer no disability in memory. Another notable exception is that, if the corpus collosum fails to develop because of some congenital anomaly, centers for language and other functions may develop in compensation on both sides of the brain. Normally, however, training transfers from one side of the brain to the other, but when the corpus collosum is impaired the subsequent training of one does not help the other side.

It is generally recognized that when a right-handed person has a cerebrovascular accident or stroke affecting the left hemisphere, he develops a paralysis on the right side of the body. Conversely, if it affects the right hemisphere, he suffers from a paralysis on the left side. Injuries of the temporal parietal area on the right side produce a disturbance of spatial perception, loss of awareness of body scheme, and loss of spatial relationships. A corresponding injury in the left side has the effect of producing the most severe disruption of language and its associated thought processes. This raises the possibility that the right hemisphere assumes a dominant role for spatial relationships and the left hemisphere a dominant role for temporal relationships. If one assumes that for the language function the temporal relationships are most crucial, then it is logical for the language function to be developed in the left hemisphere of the brain.

A change in dominance can be brought about under two pathological conditions: (1) injury to the dominant hand, or (2) injury to the dominant hemisphere of the brain. As an example, a child who is right-handed and has his right hand amputated at age 6 will become pathologically left-handed. If, 21 years later this same individual develops a tumor in the right hemisphere, which requires removal of his right hemisphere, he will probably lose the power of speech (aphasia) because the dominance had shifted to the right hemisphere. This is one example of a shift in dominance as a result of a peripheral defect, occurring only after an early change in peripheral stimulation and only after 21 years of training. Language is found in a ratio of 97 percent to 3 percent in the individual who has left hemisphere dominance. This is not true, however, in left-handed individuals. In this group, lesions in the right hemisphere in the left-handed individual need not produce an aphasia or language disability in more than 59 percent of the cases. And if there is a right hemisphere involvement, only 41 percent will be left-handed. Thus, left hemisphere dominance is more likely to be consistent, but right hemisphere dominance is not consistent with aphasia when surgery is done to the respective hemisphere.

Rasmussen (1964) found that patients in whom left-handedness was due to early brain damage were more likely to have speech in the right hemisphere. But 22 percent still had speech facility in the left side. The fact that a patient is left-handed indicates that unilateral dominance is less strongly developed and speech often tends to be bilaterally represented. When there is clinical evidence of brain injury on the left side at birth, speech is usually found to be located on the right side of the brain in two thirds of the cases.

The significance of these findings is that the dominant brain hemisphere for language is most often the left. Even in individuals who are left-handed, the left hemisphere is still very likely to be dominant for the language function. An exception to this occurs when an injury to the dominant hemisphere occurs in childhood and can be compensated for by a shift of dominance to the opposite hemisphere. While the language function in most persons is sub-served primarily by the left hemisphere, the right hemisphere has the capability for this task if the task is forced upon it. This transfer of dominance rarely occurs in adults and is usually successful only in children under the age of 8 years.

Apraxia is the inability to perform a skilled act or series of movements. There are a number of types of this disability, such as one called "ideomotor apraxia." This is the inability to perform familiar acts on verbal command or by imitation, such as making a fist or saluting or waving goodbye. Some researchers felt that apraxia resulted from a lesion of the left dominant hemisphere. In the 1920s Gerstmann described an unusual deficit associated with lesions of the major hemisphere. The parts of this syndrome, known as Gerstmann's syndrome, were (1) finger agnosia, or the inability to identify fingers on tactile stimulation; (2) loss of ability to discriminate left and right side of the body; (3) loss of ability to write (agraphia); and (4) the loss of the ability to do mathematics (acalculia).

The question has been raised as to whether the nondominant hemisphere does not have some distinctive function with respect to behavior. Neurologists, such as Brain in 1945, called attention to the fact that deficits in the right nondominant hemisphere produced impairment in visual space perception, constructional apraxia, apraxia for dressing, and inattention to one half of the visual field. This group of symptoms from both the major and the minor hemispheres, therefore, all suggest the possibility of the origin of those symptoms that are frequently found in children who have dyslexia or severe reading disability. In other words, dyslexia can occur from a dysfunction in either the major or minor hemisphere.

Furthermore, there is a question as to the role of the right hemisphere in right-handed individuals—that is, of the lesser hemisphere. Critchley (1964) suggested that the right hemisphere plays a significant role in mediating higher level language performances of the right-handed individuals, with the left hemisphere subserving more basic language processes. There are certain conclusions that can be drawn from individuals with minor or nondominant hemispheric lesions.

1. They show a greater impairment in spatial perception and memory as expressed by difficulty in following or remembering routes or by an inability to locate places on a map.
2. There is impairment in visuoconstructive activity, the so-called constructional apraxia, for example, the inability to copy or to draw a design of one's house.
3. Defects exist in visual perception and memory for nonverbal material, such as scenic representations, faces, or abstract figures.
4. Impairment in certain aspects of auditory perception and memory is more frequently encountered in individuals with right-hemispheric lesions.
5. There is motor impersistence that consists of the inability of the individual to sustain a movement that he or she has been able to initiate on verbal command, such as keeping his or her eyes closed or keeping his tongue protruding.

Each of these five points is found more frequently in individuals with minor hemispheric lesions.

Increasing evidence has been accumulated by some professionals in the educational field for the assumed correlation of certain disorders in children's language development with delayed or incomplete establishment of preferential laterality. Brain (1945) and Subirana (1961) both state, however, that poor dominance or ill-defined laterality is not a cause of language difficulty; rather, it is a concomitant symptom reflected on a parallel level. The basic deviation of brain function is responsible for both language and laterality disorders. In other words, if there is cerebral immaturity, there may be disorders of laterality and of learning.

The issue or confusion over the role of dominance was first raised by Orton in 1937. His view was that many of the delays and defects in the development of the language function may result from a deviation in the process of establishing unilateral brain superiority. This concept of hemispheric dominance was a sensation among educators and Orton's views were widely circulated. Left-handedness in cases of reading disabilities or dyslexia was frequent, and some disorder of dominance was a convenient explanation. But the answer is not so simple. There are many exhaustive tests for eye, hand, foot, and ear dominance. The theory that individuals with severe reading disability have poorly lateralized dominance may be because 20 percent of these children may have some form of brain dysfunction, which may lead to poor lateralization and poor learning. In these cases, the poor lateralization might be the result of brain dysfunction; the poor learning is associated with the dysfunction and not with crossed dominance.

It is not the loss of laterality that produces a disorder of language, but if there is a delay in the acquisition of language, most often it is accompanied by other signs of cerebral immaturity, including delayed or incomplete establishment of laterality. The anomaly of handedness is a corollary and not a cause of severe reading disabilities. There is little purpose in using one hand or patching one eye in an effort to establish dominance of one hemisphere.

Research has failed to support crossed dominance as a consistent link with reading problems. Some children with crossed dominance have no reading difficulties, while others with inconsistent laterality exhibit the entire chain of reading difficulties.

Early work by Whittey and Kopel (1936) and Johnston (1942) revealed the association between mixed hand and eye dominance with reading disability and found no correlation between anomalies of lateral dominance and reading disability. By matching a group of 50 poor readers with a control group of 50 reading achievers, Smith (1950) found no difference between them in hand, foot, ear, and eye preference.

Many blind people learning Braille use the left hand, which is most frequently the better sensory receptor. Because the right hemisphere of the brain is most often nondominant and is concerned with spatial relationships, blind persons tend to favor the left hand as their most perceptive hand when reading Braille. This may be a result of their need to feel the spacings while using their fingers to judge relationships between raised letters. The blind person rapidly reading Braille "sees" with both right and left hands and receives sensory impressions from both the right and left sides of the body at the same time. This compares with the eyes, where such bilateral stimulation is recognized as a phenomenon of retinal rivalry. Unequal retinal rivalry may lead to suppression and amblyopia, but these physiologic disturbances do not result in dyslexia. A child can recognize clues in space with one eye or two, and thus far reversals have not proven to be an abnormality of retinal rivalry.

The effect of dominance and the controlling eye can best be demonstrated by an illustration of the retinal rivalry phenomenon (see Figure 7-1).

A differential may be made between the controlling eye and the dominant eye. The dominant eye is usually the sighting or fixing eye, perhaps selected because it is optically better and therefore produces a clearer image on the retina. If the image produced by the dominant eye, however, is significantly reduced by pathology, refractive errors, or any other impediment of focusing, then there could be a transfer for visual control, and the opposite eye would become the "controlling eye." There is no immediate shift of the sighting eye, because this is a corticovisuomotor relationship that has been established by years of usage. The controlling eye can be changed by simple changes of refraction.

Reversals and translocation of letters are examples of persistent immaturity that are not peculiar to the reading disabled. These errors are notoriously common among all beginners in reading and writing. Usually, however, they are eliminated in the first 2 years of

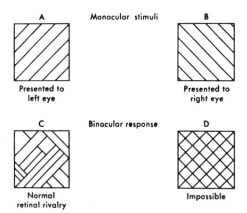

Figure 7-1. Illustration of Retinal Rivalry. In A, we expose the left eye to diagonal lines in the right-left direction. In B, we expose the right eye to diagonal lines in the left to right direction. When these stimuli are seen simultaneously, there is no fusion into a cross hatch as in D. What is really seen is an alternating degree of A and B. If ocular control is greater in one eye, more of the pattern from that eye will be similar to C. This is not dependent on dominance.

school. Yet the potential for reversals is never eliminated. The adult typist, even a professional typist, continues to make letter reversals when working at high speed or under conditions of stress and fatigue. Proofreading is another example of a persistent reversal tendency. The proofreader misses reversals and translocations in abundance, reading the words as they should be, without seeing errors because his or her mind has automatically corrected them.

The causes of reversals can be summarized as follows: (1) maturational lag, normal in children under the age of 5-years; (2) lack of auditory and visual feedback; (3) stress (usually emotional) or pressure; (4) pathological sequential disability as in parietal lobe dysfunction; and (5) delayed development of handedness and body image.

The severe reading disabled individual is not unique in making reversals but is unique in making so many for so long a time. The problems of reversal and translocation are not due to faulty dominance. The confusion can be related to the directional orientation of a symbol, in relationship to the kinesthetic feel of "making" that symbol. For instance, if one closes his or her eyes and writes the word "you" on a piece of paper held against one's forehead, one can take the card down and see that, almost certainly it has been written "uoy." We are so accustomed to writing on a surface facing the eyes that, when we write on a surface that faces away from the eyes, we automatically write as if the surface were transparent and the eyes were seeing the message. There is, then, some confusion between visual and bodily images that seems to underline some of the difficulties of directional orientation so characteristic of severely reading disabled individuals.

The following example will further emphasize and demonstrate that right and left orientation is not only a matter of dominance, but also a matter of normal relationship of visual imagery to kinesthetic imagery. Hold your palms facing you, with the forearms crossed. Keep the wrists crossed and turn the hands so that the palms face each other and lace your fingers into the corresponding interdigital spaces of the other hand. Then, with your eyes closed, have someone touch one finger. You will undoubtedly have some difficult in recognizing which finger is being touched. In fact, if someone were to touch your index finger, you would first have to start the impulse higher up in the arm and feel the impulse come down the arm and into the finger before you would know exactly which finger you were dealing with.

The more carefully one investigates handedness, the more it appears to be a continuous variable. Few adults—and even fewer children—prove to be absolutely right-handed or left-handed. It is true that if a person is right-handed, or claims to be right-handed, then he or she may be superior on the right side as compared to the left. But one cannot make the corresponding prediction if an individual states that he or she is left-handed. A large number of self-classified left-handed individuals show equal or greater preference for the use of the right hand in various activities.

As ocular dominance cannot be explained by eye anatomy, hand dominance cannot be explained by brain anatomy. There is no anatomical arrangement in the eyes themselves, or in their brain connection, that could account for the dominance of say, the right eye. There is no straightforward anatomical relationship between eye dominance and brain dominance. Shifting the controlling eye can be expected to have little effect upon hand and brain dominance.

In discussing laterality and reading problems, Orton (1937) emphasized the importance of establishing a dominant hemisphere. He claimed that engrams were formed in the associative tracts of both hemispheres, but that those in the nondominant hemisphere were not usually employed. If a clearcut dominance was not established between the two hemispheres, then the engrams of the nondominant side would be mirrorwise. Thus, attempts to change handedness perhaps might result in poor orientation and backwardness in reading.

It has been pointed out time and again that many disabled readers are left-handed or poorly lateralized insofar as hand, foot, and eye are concerned. There is a suggestion of a correlation, but it has yet to be proven what the significance of this correlation might be.

Belmont and Birch (1964) found a 10 percent rate of sinistrality in both good and disabled readers. Kinsbourne (1978) suggested that although there was no support for a causal relation with sinistrality, there might yet exist a statistical association with certain subgroups of learning disabled children. The association of mixed handedness or incomplete hand dominance with dyslexia has been documented by Ingram and Reid (1956). Less than 20 percent of normal and almost 50 percent of reading disabled 7 year olds exhibit mixed hand dominance (Harris, 1970). Thus incomplete handedness is much more strongly related to learning problems than in sinistrality.

The significance of mixed eye–hand–foot preferences is more problematical. A number of researchers have fairly conclusively demonstrated that crossed laterality has no relationship to either the diagnosis or treatment of reading problems (Rabinovitch et al., 1956; Silver, 1961). For example, Belmont and Birch (1964) found consistent eye-hand dominance in half of both average and disabled readers, with mixed eye-hand dominance being present in just under a third of both groups. Thus, most children by 5 years of age can tell the examiner which is their right and which is their left hand; by 7 years of age they can perform crossed commands. It is often not until 9 years of age that a child can identify right and left on a mirror image. Cerebral maturity and dominance are directly proportional. Children who establish right-handed tendencies early also present the earliest and best-developed signs of general psychomotor maturity. Conversely, cerebral immaturity and poorly differentiated laterality could be directly correlated. The less clearly dominance is established in a given child, the greater are the signs of his general immaturity and the more apt he is to have learning disabilities. The fact that dyslexia seems to have a genetic tendency can be explained by the fact that left-handedness too, has a genetic tendency. But left-handedness as such cannot be regarded as a simple inversion of right-handedness because there are different types of left-handedness, a genetic and a pathologic form of left-handedness. Finally, in children with poor right-left orientation, it need not only be a matter of cerebral dominance but of a relationship of visual imagery to kinesthetic imagery, sometimes known as body image.

It is agreed that severe reading disability is not more frequently present among those children who are poorly lateralized. A lack of definite lateral specialization may imply an atypical cerebral dominance, but atypical cerebral dominance is not characteristic of a large percentage of dyslexics. Severe reading disability itself may result from early brain damage or constitutional defects in maturation or retardation secondary to stress, or it may be due to a combination of these and other factors. It should be clear that the solution to problems associated with reading cannot be remediated simply by changing eye dominance or by laterality training in isolation. Rather, because of the complexity of the problem, an interdisciplinary approach that utilizes the best talent of the various educational and medical disciplines is essential.

SUMMARY

The notion of cerebral dominance owes its origin to the discovery that a loss of speech almost always results from lesions of the left hemisphere. Inevitably, this suggested a possible link with handedness and lateralization of speech due to an inborn functional pre-eminence of the left brain hemisphere. It is assumed that the position is exactly reversed in left-handers. The dominant hemisphere is accepted, with few exceptions, as being contralateral to the preferred hand.

Sufficient evidence has been accumulated to indicate that cerebral dominance and poorly defined laterality are not related to learning disorders. Right-hand preference is usually associated with left cerebral dominance, but left-hand preference does not consistently signify right cerebral hemisphere dominance. Furthermore, severe reading disability can occur as a result of a dysfunction in either the major or minor hemisphere.

REFERENCES

Benton, C., & McGann, J. Dyslexia and dominance. *Journal of Pediatric Ophthalmology,* 1969, *6,* 220.

Benton, H. Problems of cerebral dominance. *Bulletin of the Orton Society,* 1966, *16,* 38–54.

Belmont, L., & Birch, H. Auditory-visual integration in normal and retarded readers. *American Journal of Orthopsychiatry,* 1964, *34,* 852–861.

Brain, W. Speech and handedness. *Lancet,* 1945, *2,* 837.

Critchley, M. *Developmental dyslexia.* London: William Heineman Medical Books, 1964.

Gerstmann, J. Finger Agnosie und isolerte agraphia. *Zeitschrift fur die gesamte Neurologie und Psychiatrie,* 1927, *108,* 152.

Geschwind, N. Anatomical evolution of the brain. *Bulletin of the Orton Society,* 1972, *22,* 7–13.

Gordon, H. Left-handedness and mirror writing, especially among deflective children. 1921, *Brain, 43,* 313–330

Johnston, P. The relationship of certain anomalies of vision in lateral dominance to reading disability. Washington, D.C.: *Monograph for the Society for Research and Child Development,* 1942, *71,* 2.

Moreau, W. P. A case of congenital word blindness. *British Medical Journal,* 1896, *22,* 1378–1379.

Mountcastle, V. (ed.). *Interhemispheric relations and cerebral dominance.* Baltimore, Maryland: John Hopkins Press, 1962.

Orlando, C. Measures of handedness as indicators of language latrialization. *Bulletin of the Orton Society,* 1972, *22,* 14–26.

Orton, S. *Reading, writing and speech problems in children.* London: Chapman and Hall, 1937.

Penfield, W., & Roberts, L. *Speech and brain mechanisms.* Princeton, New Jersey: Princeton University Press, 1959.

Rabinovitch, R. Draw, A., Dejong, R., Ingram, W., & Witney, L. A research approach to reading retardation. In R. McIntosh and C. Hare (Eds.), *Neurology and psychiatry in childhood.* Baltimore, Maryland: Williams and Wilkinson, 1956, ch. 15.

Rasmussen, A. Laterization of cerebral speech dominance. *Journal of Neurosurgery,* 1964, *23,* 400–424.

Smith, L. A study of laterality characteristics by retarded readers and reading achievers. *Journal of Experimental Research,* 1950, *18,* 321–329.

Sperr, R. The great cerebral commissure. *Scientific American,* 1926, January, 43–52.

Subirana, A. Problems of cerebral dominance. *Logos,* 1961, *4,* 85.

Subirana, A. Relationship between handedness and language function. *Journal of Neurology,* 1964, *4,* 215–234.

Wada, J. Presentation at the 9th International Congress of Neurology. New York: *Bulletin of the Orton Society,* 1969, *19.*

Whittey, P., & Kopel, D. Factors associated with the etiology of reading disability. *Journal of Educational Research,* 1936, *29,* 449–459.

Zangwill, O. L. *Dyslexia in relation to cerebral dominance and reading disability.* Baltimore, Maryland: John Hopkins University Press, 1960.

8

Hearing and Auditory Perception

Increasing emphasis continues to be placed on the development of auditory skills in facilitating the reading process. The work of Johnson and Myklebust in 1967 clearly indicated that the auditory capacity required for reading differs from that required for speaking, while Ford (1967) found auditory-visual integration to be a significant aspect of reading ability. Of still greater significance are those skills that enable a student to sequence auditory stimuli in time. It is also important to note that our traditional concept of hearing has not always considered the varieties of individual skills that are necessary in the reading process.

There are many similarities between the visual and auditory domain. Just as there are peripheral visual factors, so there are peripheral auditory factors. Similarly, visual-perceptual as well as auditory-perceptual factors are evidenced in some learning disabilities. These perceptual factors involve the central or cerebral mechanisms of learning. Perception is distinguished from sensations and cognition. It occupies an intermediate position between simple peripheral sensations and more complex cognitional behavior.

Hearing is the sensory function that permits an organism to respond to various kinds of acoustic stimuli. The infant responds to the mother's voice, the 6-month-old child responds by turning his head to a source of sounds, a 24-month-old child responds to words and phrases, the 40-month-old child will respond to the details of a sentence, and the 5-year-old child will normally respond to other, more academic learning situations.

A variety of factors can contribute to impaired hearing, such as trauma, infection, genetic factors, and perinatal hypoxia, as a result of mechanical factors attendant on passage through the birth canal.

A comprehensive audiological evaluation answers the question of whether a hearing loss is communicatively handicapping and, therefore, educationally significant. A differential hearing evaluation allows one to answer questions that include: (1) What is the causal picture? (2) Is learning involved? (3) How much does the child hear? (4) How does he hear? (5) What course of treatment is indicated?

During the first 6 months of life as normal children progress through stages of reflex sounds and babbling, they depend upon the auditory system for feedback to establish natural language. Single-word utterances are mastered by the end of the first year of life. Those who listen to the character of the babble and to the quality of the sound produced may be aware that some children are born with normal hearing that deteriorates during the first year or two of life. All children usually utter a variety of single words by the first birthday and say simple sentences by 24 months of age. Because language development begins at birth in the normal child, hearing deficits should be addressed at this time. It is important to remember that the handicap of early childhood hearing loss is one of the most serious limitations that can befall children, since it prevents optimal development and seriously impairs relationships to the world in which they live.

The physiologic features of speech involved in peripheral hearing are frequency, rate, and intensity. Frequency is the number of vibrations per second produced by a source of sound. Human hearing is concerned with a range of sound waves between 20–20,000 Hz. Audiologists test between 125–8,000 Hz.

Intensity or loudness is the amount of energy necessary to produce a sound wave and is of importance because the intensity of consonants is weaker compared to that of vowel sounds. Rate is important because it involves the ability to resolve rapidly changing acoustical stimuli into distinctive units of complexity to identify speech sounds. The more rapidly the speech sounds are produced, the less likely is the ear able to perceive clues of a spoken word. Differences between words are more difficult to hear if the rate is increased.

Measurement of hearing can be obtained by a clinical audiologic appraisal. Two commonly employed kinds of audiologic tests are (1) those concerned with measurements of sensitivity in terms of frequency and intensity relative to stimulation by pure tones measured with air-conducted or bone-conducted stimuli, including behavioral and electrophysiological measures, and (2) tests of auditory discrimination abilities.

The speech-hearing tests are important because the child's capacities in interpreting speech are major factors in his or her ability to learn. Therefore, it is important to know not only how a child hears, but how much a child hears. Can the child distinguish and differentiate between sounds that he hears? A child who has difficulty in differentiating between sounds may be a child with a learning disability.

The importance of identifying hearing impairments in children is well-recognized by audiologists, physicians, and educators. All are recognizing the need for early detection of hearing deficits and early diagnosis in order that correctional procedures can be initiated as early as possible.

Auditory perception involves altering, attention, discrimination, processing, retrieving, sequencing of spoken language, and motor expression of speech. No listening can take place without focusing and attention to the spoken word. If a child reacts to the wrong signal or if there is too much information for the child to handle, failure might be the result.

It is of interest to note how the brain filters messages. There may be numerous voices giving messages, and at a superficial level the brain can absorb many of these stimuli. But if a single message, as an instruction, is received, the brain has the power of eliminating extraneous messages and only allowing the one to which it is alerted to filter through.

Auditory perceptual maturity may not occur until the age of seven. Since only 24 percent of children have accurate auditory discrimination by the end of the second grade, deficits in this area expose children to the risk of academic failure.

Because perceiving the complex speech code is basic to language and underlies the perception of speech (Liberman, 1967), it is important to understand what happens between the hearing of the phoneme, the understanding of speech signals, and speech perception. Also, it is complex encoding that makes the sounds of speech especially efficient as vehicles for the transmission of auditory information.

For example, a child having difficulty in spelling may write *immly* for immediately or *terote* for the word territory. Normal speech is not as simple as merely the uttering of a few disjointed words, like *ship* or *beet*. Words follow one another very rapidly in whole sentences, the listener must associate almost instantaneously in order to follow the meaning and thus gather the thought from the sentence. But just as failure may occur in visual perception, there also may be failure in auditory perception. This type of defect is expressed by the child who says, "I can hear, but I just cannot understand."

Interpreting and understanding the teacher often involves more than the acuity of hearing. To illustrate further, a child in the fifth grade who writes the essay (see the following extract) on Alexander Hamilton would normally receive a failing grade because of his spelling. However, some teachers recognizing that this child has an auditory imperception may grade the paper for its content and not for its spelling.

Financlal program full parntyement of war dept incurred by continental congress. tionpmussa and full payment of state war depts. tremhislbatse of a pound paper yenerrue saf place for publie funds sources of credit finacial agent for S.U. tremnrievog. Enactment of higher tarif for revenue and protection levyinsofar excise tax on distilled liquor.

Auditory information is received in groups of letters representing speech sounds called phonemes. A child originally hears the word as a phonemic part, and then gradually builds up the phoneme into a total word. If the child has difficulty in hearing the phoneme, then he or she could have difficulty in discriminating the entire word. Not only is hearing acuity involved, but also auditory memory. The child has to retain the whole word and discriminate the individual phonemes to contrast the words that he hears.

Auditory discrimination is the capacity to distinguish between phonemes. Certain conclusions originally summarized by Wepman (1962) with reference to auditory discrimination concluded that: (1) individuals differ in their ability to discriminate sound; (2) this ability matures until the age of 8 years; (3) slow development of auditory discrimination is correlated with poor pronunciation; and (4) that there is a positive correlation between poor discrimination and poor reading.

There are groups of children who are unable to unravel an auditory message, even though they have normal hearing. These are the children who have continuous auditory perceptive difficulty which often results in academic failure. It is not uncommon for the diagnosis of aphasia or minimal brain dysfunction to be applied to such children.

Examples of these children include those who have difficulty following a series of commands and who consistently call classmates after school to ask for the homework assignment. It is not the occasional forgetfulness, but the consistent and repeated failure to remember that makes it unusual. In the school setting, the signals given by the teacher are not carried for a sufficient length of time for such a child to understand the message.

In order for a child to compare two or more speech sounds and to make judgments as to their similarity or difference, he or she must use auditory memory. This is a much more difficult process than visual discrimination and may account for the relatively high frequency of auditory perceptual deficiencies in children with severe reading problems.

Tracking is also involved when the individual processes information presented orally. One interesting observation is that Braille reading occurs at the rate of 90 words per minute while a suggested average rate of reading for a high school senior is 250 words per minute. One other interesting observation is that the rate of thought is five times the rate of speech and good listeners utilize this time gap more efficiently than poor listeners.

Some children who have difficulty in learning do not learn simple structured rules. By testing the area of "language processing," weaknesses are identified which impair learning. Memory, both short-term and long-term, has a part in this process and directly effects the ability to learn. Memory tests are available to establish the normal function of this area and traditionally involve digit and sentence repetition. In digit repetition, digits are dictated at a rate of one per second, and then the child is asked to repeat the number of digits which were dictated. Standards have been established which indicate the number of digits which should be remembered when correlated with the age of the child. Sentence repetition, another method of testing for processing, is measured by repeating a sentence which contains a given number of words. The number of words in a sentence are standardized and correlated with age.

Language reception is also important for the identification of the source of a child's learning disability and tests, such as the Peabody Picture Vocabulary Test and the Durrell, traditionally have been administered to evaluate vocabulary and the comprehension of language.

Closely related to auditory memory is auditory sequencing, which is the recall of sounds in proper time sequence. Sentences are made up of a series of sounds presented in a sequential order. There is some suggestion that impairment in auditory sequential memory is related to reading disabilities, but there still does not exist sufficient data to make a definitive statement in this area.

The subtest of the often used ITPA for auditory sequencing provides a test for language expression. In this test an envelope, a ball, a button, a piece of chalk, and a block are used. An object is presented and the child tells all that he can about the object. Evaluation is done with reference to the detailed descriptions which the child gives. We are requiring the child to sum up, to articulate, and to categorize the objects that are in front of him or her. All of these factors are important in providing information about auditory perception.

In addition to the peripheral and perceptual aspects of spoken language, there are also the motor aspects of language. If a child of 5 years has difficulty in speaking, it is possible that he or she may have had difficulty in the earlier steps of language development; but if not, there is the possibility of his or her having a motor disability. A simple example of this difficulty would be the child who is asked to repeat, "the chair is red." The child may attempt to repeat this by saying, "a er e e." A child who has this difficulty may have had problems in discrimination, processing, reception, or motor functioning. Varying degrees of disability in any of these areas can make the child a high risk for reading disabilities.

In summary, children should be carefully monitored as they reach school age to determine if their auditory abilities equal their visual abilities. We should not make the mistake of approaching children as though they learn equally well by all systems.

REFERENCES

Ford, M. Auditory-visual and tactual-visual integration in relation to reading ability. *Perceptual Motor Skills*, 1967, *24*, 831–841.

Hardy, W. & Bordley, J. Hearing evaluation in children. *Otolaryngologica Clinica North America*, 1969, February, 3–26.

Johnson, D. & Myklebust, H. *Learning disabilities: Educational principles and practices.* New York: Grune and Stratton, 1967.

Liberman, A. Perception of the speech code. *Psychological Review*, 1967, *74*, 431–461.

Start, R., Tallal, P. Perceptual and motor deficits in language impaired children. In R. W. Keith (ed.), *Central auditory and language disorders in children.* Houston: College Hill Press, 1981, pp. 121–144.

Wepman, J. Dyslexia: Its relationship to language acquisition and concept formation. In J. Money (ed.), *Reading disability.* Baltimore: Johns Hopkins Press, 1962, pp. 179–186.

Wilkin, B. Auditory perception: Implications for language development. *Journal of Research and Development in Education*, 1969, *3* (1), 53–71.

9

Learning and Drug Therapy

Learning involves a number of highly sophisticated and complicated processes, including acquisition of information, processing of information, establishment of memory, maintenance of memory, and retrieval of information. Memory is divided into its long-term and short-term aspects, both involving enormously complex processes in the brain. Short-term memory appears to be electrical-neurological in nature, but long-term memory involves biochemical processes.

Since learning and memory seem to be composed of specific and discrete sets of processes or functions, this new view suggests to some, for example, the idea that mental retardation is not a single, all-encompassing phenomenon. Rather, it is possible to think of it in terms of defects which exist in specific areas of functions, such as acquisition of information, memory formation, or memory retention. The recent discoveries about the chemistry of the brain indicate that, if we are to understand how learning really takes place, we will have to comprehend the inordinately complicated processes of interaction between heredity, development, and environment that constantly goes on in the brain.

It seems clear that learning produces chemical changes in the brain. But one cannot understand how the brain responds to an environmental input without some understanding of its particular genetic makeup. Some human behaviors, for instance, are apparently innate, precoded or preprogrammed into the brain. Learned behavior, at this point in our knowledge, does not seem to differ greatly from innate behavior, and this suggests that the chemical processes governing both innate and learned behavior may be the same or similar.

One known fact is that experience, notably the experience of learning, demonstrably and literally changes the chemistry of the brain. Experiments involving trained and untrained rats have found both chemical and anatomical changes in the brains of the trained rats, including a heavier brain cortex, more glial cells, more enzyme activity, and a superior blood supply to the brain. Other experimental work along these lines has found that the act of learning sets a specific biochemical process into motion, which alters the protein-RNA structure of the brain in a specific way. In trained rats, new fractions of RNA appear in the nerve cells of the brain. Thus, the crucial biochemical process in learning appears to involve a change in the way the brain synthesizes protein-RNA.

A drug manufactured by a national pharmaceutical laboratory is new being clinically tested in human beings to determine its value as a performance booster. Some preliminary results indicate that it may enhance memory in presenile adults, but other reports were negative. Much more experimental work will have to be done under strict controlled conditions, before any conclusions can be reached, but it is evident now that many research chemists believe that it may soon be possible to use the results from animal experiments to increase a human being's capacity for learning through controlled use of drugs.

The implications of recent experimental work for education will remain tentative because the present knowledge of the brain and of its chemistry is still incomplete. When a coherent picture of brain chemistry does emerge, it may have enormous implications for education and for the learning process. Indeed, some feel that eventually there may be a whole arsenal of drugs, each affecting a different aspect of the learning process. It may be awesome to contemplate the educational and social consequences which could materialize. Some now think that the rate at which people learn can be greatly increased by drugs, while others foresee the human capacity to learn as being increased as well.

For those with learning disabilities, the implications for the use of "learning drugs" are equally tentative. In addition to what is still unknown about learning and the biochemical processes of the brain, too little is still known about the causes of learning disability. These are certainly all tied together to some extent, and research findings in one area may help to unravel the mysteries in the other areas. For the time being, at least, drug utilization in cases of learning disability will probably be limited to individual cases and to specific types of problems.

Recent investigations have attempted to evaluate the effects of individual drugs and dietary manipulations (Wachtel, 1981). Stimulant drugs (Dexedrine, Ritalin) have been shown to effect both learning tasks and behavioral characteristics. The mechanism for the effect appears to be related upon their ability to sustain attention.

The catecholamines are the main neurotransmitters in the brain. The amphetamines reduce hyperactivity by affecting the brain's catecholamine mechanisms. They perform this task by: (1) stimulating the release of catecholamines (dopamine and norepinephrine) from the sympathetic nerve terminals, (b) preventing re-uptake of the released catecholamines, and (c) inhibiting catecholamine breakdown by monamine oxidase.

Adamson (1979) has indicated certain principles in the use of drug therapy that should be emphasized, namely, that no drug should be prescribed without firm indications for its use, precautions for toxicity should be observed, decisions for drug use should be based on an interdisciplinary decision with subsequent careful observation by teachers and parents, drugs are an adjunct and should not be the only treatment. It is unwise to use drugs if the symptoms can be corrected by other means, such as remediation by social, familial, educational, or emotional methodology. Monitoring of blood levels for some drugs is critical since these drugs can effect haematopoietic mechanisms that may precipitate leukopenia and agranulocytosis.

It is important to recognize that not one drug is universally indicated. In discussing therapeutic intervention of drugs in the learning problems of children, it should be stressed that drugs ought not be used empirically in all cases of learning disability or hyperactivity. There are, however, three groups of children who *may* benefit. First, there are the children who have minimal neurological signs (brain damage) and positive EEG findings. A child in this category may be helped by a drug such as Dilantin. The next group of children consists of those who are behaviorally disturbed. Here tranquilizers may help in the child's treatment with the most often prescribed tranquilizers being Thorazine and Valium. The third group of children who may be responsive to drug therapy is composed of those who are hyperactive and for whom Ritalin may be generally beneficial. Again, caution must be exercised as drug therapy should only be considered when traditional methodology has failed or is ineffective.

A drug must be designated for a specific reason. For example, psychostimulants as a means of increasing attention and controlling hyperactivity with Ritalin and amphetamines being the most frequently used. If there is a demonstrable convulsive aspect associated with the learning disability, then mysoline, dilantin and phenobarbitol may be considered. The choice of drug with dosage and possible complications is well described by Adamson (1979).

Other methods of therapy classified as controversial are mentioned here but with the caution that their acceptance has not been proven.

Orthomolecular therapy in learning disabilities is the use of high doses of multivitamins and the avoidance of food additives. Committees of the Academy of Science and of the Academy of Pediatrics have found no justification for this megavitamin therapy as a treatment in the learning disabled child.

Biofeedback procedures incorporate the use of electrical and mechanical devices and can be used in the management of educational problems in children. Feedback by bioelectrical responses to control respiration in an attempt to modify hyperactivity has been suggested (Simpson & Nelson, 1974) but again substantial proof as a treatment procedure is just in a beginning stage.

Feingold (1975) suggested that food additives could be responsible for hyperactivity and learning disabilities. However, limited well-controlled studies by Conners (1980), Williams (1978), and Stare (1980) appear to support the view that there is little evidence of a relationship of food additives to learning disabilities. The National Advisory Committee on Hyperkinesis stipulated the following objections to the Feingold (1975) claims:

1. There were no controls
2. Percent improvement varied with the presentation
3. Placebo effect was not considered
4. No objective measures of change were employed
5. Observer was not blind to treatment

Cott (1971) suggested that many of the symptoms of the hyperactive child were secondary to hypoglycemia and Dunn (1976) reported a study of 144 children with learning disability in which a five-hour glucose tolerance test revealed that 72 percent of this group showed some degree of abnormal carbohydrate metabolism (Leisman, 1976).

It becomes apparent that no drug should be used without some firm indication that its use may be helpful. Even though most poor readers do not show improvement with drug therapy, some do. Furthermore, it is hoped that when a drug is used, the doses will become progressively smaller until there can be a discontinuance of it. This occurs when the child is able to rely upon himself rather than upon drugs for successful attention and controlled hyperactivity in class and home settings.

In discussing hyperactivity in children, one must be careful to differentiate between hyperactivity and the results of ordinary parental permissiveness. There are a number of young children who are hyperactive and restless. They are demanding, have temper tantrums, and show short attention spans for the things they do not like. The parents, if they make no effort to discipline the child, go along with their every demand and whim; the child, in turn, remains in a preschool stage, retaining an attitude that is characteristic for preschool children. After such children get into the upper grades in school, they have increasing difficulty. When the teacher begins to set limits on their behavior, these children become disciplinary problems. This type of immature impulsiveness does not usually disappear. As a result, many children do not learn well and do not do satisfactory school work because they have never been required to discipline themselves (see Chapter 5).

The use of drugs to control such undisciplined children is often not recommended. Where only self-discipline can permanently change the behavior of such children, the use of drugs as a substitute only delays the cure. In fact, one should never try to prescribe drug therapy for a child whose symptoms might stem from a correctable social, familial, biological, or interpersonal disturbance. The use of drugs without vigorous efforts to eliminate these other etiological factors should be avoided.

The group of drugs known as phenothiazines may produce what is perceived by adults as improvement. There is increasing and compelling evidence, however, that phenothiazines and, similarly, tranquilizers actually depress the learning function. The child may appear to improve because he or she is quieter, but there is the possibility of a depression of intellect. These tranquilizers are recommended for use only when the child is extremely disruptive and when he or she has not responded to the stimulant medications.

A most frequently used instrument to monitor behavioral response to medication is the Connnors Abbreviated Teachers Rating Scale in which a score from 0 (not at all) to 3 (very much) is applied to the following 10 items:

1. restless/overactive
2. excitable, impulsive
3. disturbs other children
4. short attention span
5. fidgety
6. distractible
7. easily frustrated
8. cries often/easily
9. mood lability
10. temper tantrums/unpredictable behavior.

Total scores range from 0 to 30, with 15 being two standard deviations above the mean.

Drug therapy should not be sought lightly by parents. Drugs should be prescribed only where they will help the child, not to appease the parents. The most common side effects of drug therapy are loss of appetite, insomnia, irritability, sadness, nausea, headaches, cramps, and jitters. Once undertaken, drug therapy should be guarded. If the dosage has been pushed to the point where side effects occur and there is still doubt as to whether or not the drug is effective, then it is not effective and should be discontinued.

As incredible as it seems, children in primary grades (ages 7, 8, 9) are already demonstrating symptoms of drug overdose. In such cases, their learning problems are the result of drug experimentation and usage. For them, drug abuse is a means of withdrawing from school problems or a means of challenging and defying parents, the teacher, or the society in which they are failures. For some students it may be the lure of a promised "mind expansion" that will solve their learning difficulties.

Doubtless there are many other reasons why children resort to drugs. Whether they do so because of academic failure of whether academic failure results from their drug abuse, these children create classroom problems of great magnitude. If the experimentation with drugs by children in the lower grades continues to grow, we may be confronted with large numbers of cases of learning disability that have been induced by drug usage.

In children, profound behavioral changes result from a psychological dependence on drugs. The use of "hard drugs" (opium, heroin, morphine, cocaine, and certain barbiturates that are depressants) show effects that range from severe depression and irrational behavior to overexcitement, rage, and uncontrolled violence in the absence of the drug. Some drugs, on the other hand, produce completely apathetic children. Where a physiological dependence has been established, the absence of the drug leads to a wide range of familiar "withdrawal" symptoms, such as perspiration, dilated pupils with blurred vision, and nausea. Because these drugs are illegal, various aspects of antisocial behavior are associated with the attitudes and actions of the users.

Because many important biochemical, neurophysiological, and general physiological factors are involved in the learning process, it should be evident that drugs and chemical compounds represent a significant and potentially critical intervention in that process. Where drug use is illicit and self-administered, the prognosis is not good for learning in the classroom situation. For a number of problems associated with learning and with learning disability, however, therapeutic drug intervention may be beneficial. This involves the use of carefully selected drugs, prescribed, administered, monitored, and evaluated by the appropriate medical practitioner.

REFERENCES

Adamson, W., & Adamson, K. *Handbook for specific learning disabilities.* New York: Gardner Press, 1979.

Conners, C. K. *Food additives and hyperactive children.* New York: Plenum Press, 1980.

Cott, A. Orthomuscular approach to the treatment of learning disabilities. *Schizophrenia,* 1971, *3,* 95–105.

Dunn, P. Orthomolecular therapy: Implications for learning disability. In G. Leisman (ed.), *Basic visual processes and learning disability.* Springfield, Illinois: Charles C. Thomas, 1976, pp. 359–370.

Feingold, B. Hyperkinesis and learning disabilities linked to artificial food flavors and colors. *American Journal of Nursing*, 1975, *75*, 797–803.

Leisman, G. *Basic visual processes and learning disability*. Springfield, Illinois: Charles C. Thomas, 1976.

Simpson, D. & Nelson, A. Attention training through breathing control to modify hyperactivity. *Journal of Learning Disabilities*, 1974, *7*, 274–283.

Stare, F. J., Whelan, E. M., & Sheridan, M. Diet and hyperactivity: Is there a relationship? *Pediatrics, 1980, 66*, 521.

Wachtel, R. *Drugs, diet, learning, and behavior.* Unpublished presentation at the Symposium on Learning Disabilities, John F. Kennedy Institute, Baltimore, Maryland, February, 1981.

Williams, J., Cram, D.M., Tausig, F. T., et al. Relative effects of drugs and diet on hyperactive behaviors: An experimental study. *Pediatrics, 1978, 61*, 811.

10

Genetics and Reading Disabilities

Genetic inheritance is determined by information generated in the chromosomes. Forty-six chromosomes are estimated to contain 20,000 to 40,000 different gene pairs, which are subject to variation as a result of mutations of structure. Abnormalities in recombination, translocation, and random distribution can further increase these variations. Few diseases are either totally genetic or entirely environmental in their pathogenesis. Genetic information can be conveyed by a single reaction that may be under the control of a specific genetic locus. Cell function is under extensive genetic control, and mutation of a single gene can result in a structural alteration of the cell, and therefore, the ability of the cell to carry out a single primary chemical reaction can be abolished.

The gene consists of protein material containing deoxyribonucleic acid (DNA) that forms a template on which other nucleic acid molecules of precise structure are synthesized. There are two kinds of nucleic acid: deoxyribonuclei (DNA) and ribonucleic (RNA). They are chemically similar but functionally different.

Chromosome aberrations responsible for congenital anormalies were unrecognized in man until recently. These aberrations were not understood until the invention of light microscopy, which permitted the human eye to visualize what had been foreseen 35 years earlier by clinical observation. By tissue cultivation where a sufficient number of cells are stopped in mitosis by addition of colchicine, a sufficient number of metaphases can be observed on a microscopic slide.

In man, the primordial germ cell contains 2 sets each of 23 chromosomes, each set inherited from one of the two parents. Except for the XY sex pair in males, each member of a set has its homologue in the other set. At the first division, homologues "recognize" each other and form pairs which exchange genetic material. At fertilization, two cells, each with one set of single chromosomes, fuse to form a zygote, at which time the diploid number of chromosomes of the species is restored.

A pictorial display in which an attempt is made to pair homologous chromosomes and to arrange them according to size is called a karyotype. Chromosomes are studied most commonly at the metaphase stage because they are more easily distinguished at that time.

Every chromosome in a normal set can be assigned to one of seven groups labeled A-G, in order of decreasing size. Chromosomal aberrations may be manifested by changes in the structure or number of chromosomes, or both. Variations in size, shape, or position, affect multiple systems.

On reviewing the karyotype, one would not expect to see any abnormality that would be specific for a reading disability. Translocation and other abnormalities would lead to greater malformations than would be found in a child with only auditory or visual memory defects. Evidence for the genetic inheritance of dyslexia, therefore, must be obtained from other examinations involving parents, siblings, and twin pedigree studies of the individual case history.

Reading disability has been the object of study by investigators from various disciplines, including neurologists, pediatricians, educators, and most recently, the experimental psychologist. Even though heredity has been cited as a cause for some cases of reading disability, there has been little participation in this research area by the geneticist. The two principle reasons for this have been (1) the difficulty in finding adequate tangible evidence that is suitable for genetic analysis, and (2) the problem of reaching agreement on some definitions of reading disability.

The syndrome of reading disability can be fragmented into many clinical and genetic conditions. Childs (1979) has cited mental retardation as an example. Some cases are due to trauma or infection, others to gene disease and chromosomal abnormalities. Childs shows a phenotypic heterogeneity in reading disabilities which include subtypes, namely: (1) visual spatial, (2) dysphonetics, (3) language disorder, (4) auditory memory, and (5) visual perceptual.

Since the control of human behavior is a genetic function and reading is a behavioral function, we may look at the evidence for reading disability as a genetic problem. The evidence established thus far involves the following areas: (1) pedigree or family history, (2) the presence of learning disabilities in monozygotic and dizygotic twins, (3) the likelihood that a genetically determined reading disability will persist through a lifetime, (4) the determination of biochemical and chromosomal aberrations, and (5) the presence of characteristically abnormal visually evoked responses in family pedigrees.

Several studies of reading disabled children have included the family history of reading disability as one of several factors under investigation. Among those studies are investigations by Eustis (1947), Symmes and Rapoport (1972), Ingram et al. (1970), and Rutter and Yale (1975), all of which found a high incidence of reported reading disability in the families of subjects under study.

Naidoo (1972) studied the relationship of familial history to other features of reading disability to determine if different types of reading disorders existed, and to determine if features of a subgroup might support etiology. These studies did show a high incidence of reading problems in the families of children with reading problems.

Critchley (1963) has suggested that it is rare to find a child with reading problems who does not have a family with one or more similarly afflicted members. Bryant and Patterson (1962) assert that, in many cases, probably more than half of their probing interviews would reveal that other family members have also shown a reading disability. Although not necessarily a convincing argument for the genetic basis of reading disability, Hallgren in 1950 employed genetic statistical techniques in his research, with some convincing results. While an important genetic component of the problem certainly seems to suggest, although the evidence is not yet conclusive, that genetic defect is basic to some reading disability.

Opposed to the idea of the genetic origin of reading problems is the fact that no chemical or other objective proof that such problems are genetically determined has yet been put forward, nor would one expect a biochemical change in a dominant disorder. At a conference at the California Institute of Technology on the "Biological

Basis of Human Behavior,'' Childs (1979) discussed the genetics of reading disability and indicated that chromosomal abnormalities were not present in these cases.

One of the intriguing problems here is the fact that many of the handicaps which result in defects in the ability to process visual or auditory information, or to coordinate and integrate both of these processes, are found in most young children who are just beginning to read. In a child with a reading disability, however, these defects persist sometimes for months, sometimes for years, and sometimes for a lifetime. Thus, the question arises as to whether or not it is fair to label as "genetic" a handicap present in most children, but one for which most can learn to compensate.

The difficulty in dealing with this question may be seen in the early work of Silver and Hagin (1964). They examined 24 persons whom they had observed 10 years earlier as cases of reading disability, and whom they retested, using the same battery of tests. In addition to reading, their methods included testing visual-motor, auditory, and tactile functions. The results indicated that of the 24 subjects, 15 had since become good readers while 9 had not. More significantly, they found that the majority still showed the same deficiencies in the nonreading functions that they had shown 10 years earlier.

In 1962, Bryant and Patterson pointed out that the hormonal imbalance, suggested by the feminine appearance of some boys with reading disability, may or may not be genetically determined. Maturational lag or the slower development of certain cerebral areas (as a genetically influenced development) may be present in many cases of children with reading disability who are immature in size and appearance and who perform like much younger children.

In looking at a genetic phenotype to submit for analysis, various factors involved in reading must be considered. These include: performance, oral and silent reading, spelling, word meaning, perception and spatial patterns, memory for unrelated items, perceptual speed, and other cognitive functions. The development of reading skill is dependent in part on the cultural and emotional climate of the immediate family. Thus, if uncles, aunts, and cousins show evidences of reading disability in the same frequency as that found in the index family, the likelihood or origin of the reading problem in cultural or emotional factors is reduced.

Boder (1968) described three groups of children: those defective in phonetic skills, those deficient in visual perception, and a third group, particularly resistant to treatment, showing deficiencies characteristic of both of the first two groups. The source of the defects in all three of these groups could be familial, and Boder suggests that the siblings show the same deficiencies. Three patterns of deficiency were found by Ingram (1960). One group of children had visual-spatial problems, a second group had difficulty in integrating visual and auditory stimuli, while a third group had trouble comprehending words or sentences and in recalling appropriate words to express ideas. Because of the diversity of the symptomatology of all of these cases, it is just not likely that the genes would be the same for all of them. Critchley (1963) feels that to blame some environmental factor for learning disability is not likely to be correct since the evidence, in many cases, goes back from generation to generation.

The evidence for a genetic cause for specific reading disability was first noted because of the familial aggregations of cases of specific reading disability; the conclusion was made that there must be a hereditary form of it. The data favoring this hypothesis were of three kinds: (1) family history and pedigree analysis, (2) concordance of single-ovum twins, and (3) other characteristics.

One of the difficulties in pedigree analysis is that there may be one sibling who may have a similar disability, and it may appear that the parents or relatives have had a similar disability. Frankly, however, few investigators have examined the parents, relatives, and siblings of the child with the reading disability. The fact that a family group has many instances of learning disability does not prove a genetic origin. It may be accounted for by the common cultural environment experienced by members of the family.

The genetic contribution to learning disabilities is imprecise but case studies by numerous authors suggest evidence for a genetic predisposition. In a review by Finucci (1978), twin, family, and pedigree studies convincingly demonstrated the familial nature of reading disorders. When familial patterns were examined, no single mode of transmission explained all patterns. She felt that tests of specific genetic hypotheses should be done only on the families of subjects demonstrating a similar cluster of characteristics.

One major genetic study done by Hallgren (1950), examined 116 disabled readers and discovered 160 secondary cases in their families. Hallgren did extensive physical examinations and gave informal reading and spelling tests to the parents and to other adult relatives. He concluded that primary dyslexia is a dominant characteristic. Hallgren also found no consistent relationship between reading disabilities and handedness.

Hallgren (1950) listed the following as his criteria for a positive diagnosis of specific reading disability: (1) difficulties in learning to read and write; (2) proficiency in reading and writing during the first years of school definitely below the average of the class the child attended; (3) a definite discrepancy between proficiency in reading and writing and in other school subjects; and (4) a definite discrepancy between proficiency in reading and writing and the child's general intelligence.

Hermann has studied 45 sets of twins, of whom at least one twin had a reading disability. Twelve pairs of these twins were one-egg (monozygotic) or identical twins, and in all twelve pairs both twins showed identical disability. Thirty-three sets of these twins were two-egg (dizygotic) or nonidentical. Nineteen of these sets of two-egg twins were of the same sex, but in only four sets did both twins have reading disability. Fourteen sets were opposite-sex twins and in only seven sets did both twins have reading disability. Thus, in the one-egg twins there was a 100 percent concordance of disability, while in the two-egg twins there was only 33 percent concordance. These findings would *indicate* that dyslexia may be genetically determined and not dependent on environmental influences. It is commonly observed that any genetically determined characteristic persists for life, while variations due to developmental change disappear in time, and those due to injury may be overcome by healing processes. If there is a genetic cause of some cases of reading disability, then one must realize that they are never outgrown and the appropriate treatment is one that rearranges the environment so as to allow the affected person to tolerate his disability. This relates directly to the work of Margaret Rawson (1968), who interviewed and followed patients who had reading problems for 20 years. She found that, although the educational attainments of these people were no less than those of normal readers, many of them continued to find reading and spelling an embarrassing task.

In summary, there are some reasons for believing that reading disability can be genetically determined. Familial groupings of cases do exist. The observation of reading difficulties in twins, especially identical twins, is strongly suggestive of a genetic origin. The persistence of the reading deficiency characteristic into adult life in some persons is also compatible with the genetic hypothesis.

Before a genetic etiology can be proved, there must be much better evidence of heredity and the possibility of genetic heterogeneity. A child may have different genes that provoke different symptoms, such as finger agnosia, memory difficulty, or a visual-perceptual difficulty. Yet, each one of these difficulties may produce a learning disability.

The appropriate use of genetic analysis, together with the broadening of the set of phenotype characteristics to be tested, should include neurophysiological and biochemical attributes and should tell us whether or not reading disabilities are genetically determined, how many hereditary types there are, and perhaps the frequency of the genes that cause them. This mode of attack upon the problem of reading disability may be of questionable importance or, even, merely academic. Since we are not going to have selective breeding of human beings, we are still going to have to try to educate the child who is unable to achieve, who becomes frustrated, and who may be resentful and disturbed.

Children with reading disabilities can succeed, as evidenced by individuals, such as Winston Churchill, Harvey Cushing, Thomas Edison, Albert Einstein, Paul Ehrlich, George Patton, Auguste Rodin, and Woodrow Wilson, all of whom were classified as "dyslexics."

REFERENCES

Boder, E. Developmental dyslexia: A diagnostic approach based on three atypical reading patterns. *Developmental Medicine and Child Neurology*, 1973, *15*, 663–687.

Bryant, N. & Patterson, R. *Reading disability: Part of a syndrome of neurological functioning*. Unpublished paper presented at International Reading Association, Newark, Delaware, 1962.

Childs, B. *Biological basis of human behavior*. Pasadena, California Institute of Technology, 1964.

Childs, B. & Finucci, J. The genetics of learning disabilities. In R. Porter and M. O'Connor (eds.), *Human genetics: Possibilities and realities.* New York: Excerpta Medica, 1979, pp. 359–376.

Critchley, M. The problem of developmental dyslexia. *Proceedings of the Royal Society of Medicine,* 1963, *56,* 209–211.

Eustis, R. Specific reading disability. *New England Journal of Medicine,* 1947, *237,* 243–249.

Finucci, J. Progress in learning disabilities. In H. Myklebust (ed.), *Progress in learning disabilities* (vol. IV). New York: Grune and Stratton, 1978, pp. 41–64.

Hallgren, B. Specific dyslexia (congenital word blindness): A clinical and genetic study. *Acta Psychiatrica Neurologica Supplement 65,* 1950.

Hermann, K. *Reading disability: A medical study of word blindness and related handicaps.* Springfield, Illinois: Charles C. Thomas, 1959.

Ingram, T. Pediatric aspects of specific developmental dysphasia, dyslexia, and dysgraphia. *Cerebral Palsy Bulletin,* 1960, *2,* 254–277.

Ingram, T., Mason, A. & Blackburn, I. A retrospective study of 82 children with reading disability. *Developmental Medicine and Child Neurology,* 1970, *12,* 271–281.

Rawson, M. *Developmental language disability: Adult accomplishments of dyslexic boys.* Baltimore: Johns Hopkins Press, 1968.

Rutter, M. & Yule, W. The concept of specific reading retardation. *Journal of Child Psychology and Psychiatry and Applied Disciplines,* 1975, *16,* 181–197.

Silver, A., & Hagin, R. Specific reading disability: Followup studies. *American Journal of Orthopsychiatry,* 1964, *34,* 95–102.

Symmes, J., & Rapoport, J. Unexpected reading failure. *American Journal of Orthopsychiatry,* 1972, *42,* 82–91.

11

The Complexity of the Reading Problem

The ability to read is increasingly recognized as a basic human right. At present, nearly one-fifth of the world's adult population, some 800 million men and women, are functionally illiterate. Despite a significant decline in the literacy rate over the past 25 years, the rapid growth of world population has caused an actual increase in the number of illiterates since 1950.

Even with the high level of educational development in the United States, the issue of illiteracy is of great importance for our country.

Dr. Ernest Boyer, keynoting an International Literacy Conference (1978), quoted Professor Ted R. Kilty's fascinating study of the cultural complexity of language (Kilty, 1978). Dr. Kilty found that a driver's license manual is written at a sixth grade reading level; directions on a gelatin box are at a seventh grade level; and frozen dinners are at an eighth grade level. A tenth grade reading level is required to follow instructions on an aspirin bottle. An insurance policy requires a twelfth grade reading ability while college level ability is required to comprehend an apartment lease. The Harris Survey of 1970 found 23 million Americans unable to read or write at a minimal level of competence and present reports estimate that over 50 million adults are functionally illiterate.

Ernest L. Boyer (International Literacy, 1978) once observed that the illiteracy rate climbs alarmingly when we turn to the plight of minorities, to inner city and rural dwellers, and to those in the lowest paying job categories. Nearly a quarter of our minority population has inadequate basic reading and writing skills. Eight percent of our population cannot successfully complete an application for a driver's license; 11 percent have difficulty with an application for a personal bank loan; and 34 percent fail to complete an application for Medicaid. A man or woman whose earnings are below poverty level is four times as likely to be illiterate as his or her better paid counterparts.

One only has to focus on the impact of reading disabilities on the Department of Defense (DOD) to see the magnitude of the illiteracy problem. The DOD reports that poor reading ability among many enlisted personnel has a negative impact on the effective performance of their duties and career advancement. Furthermore, poor readers, who sometimes also have motivational or attitudinal problems, tend to be discharged prematurely since many cannot complete basic training requirements. Finally, increased costs result from the illiteracy problem, including the investment in personnel who are prematurely discharged and the resulting reduction in operational effectiveness among the service units.

The services are so concerned about this illiteracy problem that they spend over 3 million dollars annually on their remedial programs and have committed over 8 million dollars to make reading materials easier to comprehend. The DOD reports that some progress has been made but that the overall illiteracy problem persists because current efforts to correct the illiteracy problem have not been totally effective.

The same gloomy information has been reported at various times by the private sector, vocational and rehabilitation programs, and the penal system.

The disturbing and amazing fact is that educators *know* how to solve this illiteracy problem. Reading specialists know how to teach most people to read. Our problem is not that we do not know what to do. Our problem is how to get this knowledge down to the classroom, the teacher, the student, the tutor, and the tutee.

In 1972, The Johns Hopkins University hosted an interdisciplinary seminar wherein the participants from 12 professional organizations concerned with literacy were asked to define severe reading disabilities, to report what their organizations were doing about it, and to decide how the groups could work together (Johns Hopkins Reading Disability Symposium, 1972). After two days of discussion, the meeting terminated because the professionals could not even agree on what they were talking about. It appears that professionals spend so much time and energy defending their positions and guarding their turf that they have little energy and time left for working together for their avowed purpose.

Schiffman, (1979b), in an interim basic skills task force reported that few federally funded programs had any communication or interaction with each other. Each agency had the tendency to follow its own legislated mandate with its designated constituents and made little attempt to interact with the others.

To complicate matters, the various professional organizations and related areas of psychology, medicine, and education often view the field from their special interest. Similar differences appeared when discussing the area with individuals, since each so-called "expert" usually represented only one of the disciplines.

Recognizing this lack of professional cooperation, several national and regional legislative actions concerned with literacy called for interdisciplinary coordination and cooperation. They include:

1. Title II of the Elementary and Secondary Education Act of 1965 (Basic Skills Improvement) Basic Skills Acts, which calls for the establishment of

> . . . a systematic strategy for improving basic skills instruction in the local district which provides for the planning and implementation of comprehensive basic skills instructional programs at the school building level. The school level program shall address the needs of all students and shall utilize, in a coordinated fashion, resources available from all Federal, State, and local sources. Teachers, administrators, and parents shall be involved in the development of the comprehensive school level programs.

In support of this legislation, in 1978–1979 the United States Office of Education (USOE) Steering Committee for Basic Skills Coordination engaged in a detailed study of the problems of coordination among education programs for children, youth, and adults who were assisted by federal legislation. They reported that one of their most serious problems was that each piece of federal education legislation had been developed to meet the needs of a specific population. That same legislation, in many instances, mandates coordination across programs. The obvious question is how to maintain the integrity of each program and yet accomplish needed coordination.

2. Title I of the Elementary and Secondary Act of 1965 states in Section 129:

> It is the intent of the Congress to encourage, whenever feasible, the development for each educationally deprived child participating in a program under this title of an individualized educational plan (maintained and periodically evaluated), agreed upon jointly by the local educational agency, the teacher, a parent or guardian of the child, and when appropriate, the child.

Based on this section of the legislation, each local education agency is urged to develop a personalized educational plan (PEP) for each participating Title I student. The plan (PEP) should draw upon services such as those provided by the school psychologist, guidance counselor, reading teacher, health services personnel, speech and hearing specialists, and curriculum and resource specialists. In addition, the local education agency may wish to have those who are involved in the development of the PEP sign it upon completion and approbation. This does not indicate that the PEP is a legal document, but only that those involved are aware of the plan and their responsibilities in making it successful. Since approximately 83 percent of Title I instructional programs involve some aspect of literacy, this action will have great impact on reading teachers and other professionals at the local building site.

3. Public Law 94-142, the Education of All Handicapped Children Act (see Chapter 13), mandates that special educational services should be extended to all children with learning problems through the efficient delivery of coordinated and effective multidisciplinary and interdisciplinary services designed to meet individual needs, regardless of the category of difficulty or disability or of the nature of the causative problems. The key words again are "cooperative and effective multidisciplinary and interdisciplinary services." Although addressing all areas of special education, PL 94-142 has great implications for the professional concerned with literacy.

The Second Annual Report to Congress on the implementation of PL 94-142 (1980) indicated that 1,281,379 children, ages 3−21 years, were served under PL 83-13 and PL 94-142 in the learning disabled handicapping condition.

The areas of *basic reading skills* and *reading comprehension* are two of the seven areas of functioning that are considered in determining the existence of a specific learning disability. A national survey of individualized educational programs for handicapped children reports that about 63 percent of handicapped children are, according to their IEPs (see Chapter 13) receiving special educational services in reading and in oral or written English. By the time students are at the 13 to 15 year age level, some 73 percent of them will receive special education assistance in reading, writing or speaking. In other words, the older the age group, the greater the emphasis on reading.

4. In this same vein of interdisciplinary cooperation, the Appalachian Regional Commission (Schiffman, 1979a), in identifying its human resources goals for the future, stated:

> It is agreed that the need exists for a new partnership in basic skills joining many groups: medical, paramedical and educational agencies; industry and labor, public and private agencies; voluntary and church organizations, community and ethnic groups; manpower and training agencies; and especially the family.

Finally, a former United States commissioner of education developed, with the chief state school officers, a basic skills agreement preamble (1979) and two memoranda of understanding between the United States Department of Education and the United States Department of Commerce (1979a), and between the United States Department of Education and the United States Department of the Navy, (1979b).

In the former document (11979a), the chief state school officers and the United States Commissioner of Education agreed to work together in the following ways to strengthen basic skills instruction.

(1) The State agrees to develop an individualized statewide basic skills improvement plan or to expand its existing plan. The statewide basic skills plan will include the following:

- Identification of the areas in which basic skills improvements are needed
- A clear statement of short- and long-range objectives
- A specific plan to achieve these objectives including a description of the way state and federal programs will be coordinated
- An evaluation plan to determine if objectives have been met
- A clear description of the way nonpublic schools will be included in the plan

(2) The state and the federal government agree to work together to ensure that grants under the nationally funded basic skills programs (Part A of Title II) and the Achievement Testing Program (Title IX) are consistent with the statewide plan. The State will review applications for grants under these programs to ensure that they support the state basic skills plan.

(3) The federal government agrees to coordinate the efforts of its many programs which influence state basic skills activities.

This last point is extremely significant if any attempt to develop a coordinated effort is to succeed.

The purpose of the memorandum of understanding between the Department of Health, Education and Welfare, U. S. Office of Education, and the Department of the Navy is to establish departmental/agency functions in administering an Interagency Agreement for an experimental test of a program designed to build vocationally relevant literacy skills. The purpose of the memorandum of understanding between the United States Office of Education and the Department of Commerce is to establish departmental/agency functions in administering an interagency agreement for a pilot demonstration project in literacy improvement designed to increase the ability of the private sector to offer upward mobility opportunities and hire the unemployed.

This innovative approach to interagency cooperation is exciting and supportive of any coordinative effort.

Of course, the federal government and regional commissions cannot legislate "coordination and cooperation" forever without really bringing about real understanding. In fact, that may be the reason that "mainstreaming" is not as effective as its proponents had predicted. Education does not have an enviable record in the area of "individualization" and mainstreaming is simply good individualization of instruction with legal teeth.

Many professionals in the past have been involved in futile attempts to build bridges of communication and cooperation among the various disciplines concerned with the severely reading disabled child. Maybe they have failed because of semantic difficulties, but one suspects this failure is greatly due to each discipline's resistance, possibly unconscious, to encroachments of other professions. Somehow, though, professionals will have to learn to work together. Mainstreaming, decreased funding, and the previously mentioned federal laws demand cooperation and a "cease and desist" to duplication of efforts.

Fortunately, when coordinators of federal programs who are

interested in literacy meet to discuss reading programs without worrying about which legislative act is responsible for the funding, they find that the successful sites contain some common principles and action steps (see Table 11-1 in the Appendix, p. 135).

SUMMARY OF READING QUESTIONNAIRES

During the 1979–1980 school year, 1375 professionals, who were attending selected reading and learning disabilities conferences around the country, were asked to evaluate their local school reading programs with respect to these identified principles and action steps (see Table 11-1 in the Appendix, p. 135). Eight hundred ninety-five elementary teachers (grades 1–6), 169 middle school teachers (grades 5–8), and 311 secondary teachers (grades 7–12) voluntarily completed the questionnaire. Although this was not a completely accurate sample nor a recommended sampling procedure, the responses do give, however, some indication of the "state of the art" (see Table 11-1 in the Appendix, p. 135).

The literature consistently reports that skilled teachers make the real difference in successful reading programs. Although the number of courses taken does not guarantee competency in any area, it does reveal some valuable information.

Table 11-2 (see Appendix, p. 136), reports:

1. Eight percent of the teachers reported that they have had a maximum of three graduate courses in reading; 838 teachers (61 percent) had obtained a graduate degree with a major in reading.
2. This alarming data reveals that only 4 percent and 2 percent of the teachers, respectively, have taken courses in learning disabilities or language development. (If one believes that reading is an integral part of language arts, a continuation of this trend cannot be justified.)
3. On a positive note, over three-fourths of the professionals had some academic training in reading diagnosis.

In Table 11-3 (see Appendix, p. 137) it is encouraging to see that 79 percent of the reading teachers' salaries are provided by nonfederal funds. In view of existing and projected cutbacks in federal funding, it is extremely important for the local sites to support reading personnel and programs.

Analyzing the role of the reading teacher from the data in

Table 11-3, one finds a wide variation of duties. Forty-one percent of the teachers work with small instructional groups. It is surprising that this percentage is not higher since this is the reading teacher's traditional responsibility. Less than one-fifth of the reading teachers reported that their major responsibility is to act as a consultant or resource person for classroom teachers, and only 19 percent conduct teacher education programs. Approximately three-fourths of these teacher education programs are conducted after school, a practice that is of questionable value.

Many specialists believe that the major remediation program takes place in the regular classroom. This concept will be increasingly supported with the full fruition of the "mainstream" philosophy, although who will be responsible for helping to individualize the instructional program is a source of some speculation.

Table 11-4 (see Appendix, p. 138) shows that more than 40 percent of the reading teachers are involved with instructional work with pupils "more than 2 years delayed in reading" while 23 percent work with pupils "less than 2 years delayed in reading." This two-year figure constantly crops up both in practice and the literature as a magic "cut off."

It is interesting to note that 4 percent of the teachers work with achieving pupils, a percentage that will probably increase with the expanding interest with the high achiever.

Table 11-5 (see Appendix, p. 139) reveals an interesting trend. Years ago, few remedial reading programs even mentioned working with primary children, attributing their problems to their being "late bloomers." According to the survey, 35 percent of instruction is directed to K−3 pupils. Undoubtedly, this greater emphasis on early identification and remediation will continue to increase.

It is also important to note from the survey that over 90 percent of the reading teacher's time is spent with less than 10 percent of the school's students. This is additional evidence that the major responsibility of reading instruction lies in the hands of regular classroom teachers.

Questions 3 and 4 in Table 11-5 indicate how little involvement the reading teacher has with the special education teacher and with the interdisciplinary diagnostic and treatment teams. Even when the reading teacher is involved with exceptional children, he or she usually works alone.

As is to be expected, in Table 11-6 (see Appendix, p. 140)

reading teachers employ a variety of remediation techniques with only about one-fourth specifying a pedagogical procedure. Interestingly enough, over one-half of the professionals reported a continued emphasis on the development of word recognition skills. According to Table 11-6, this is to be expected since many identified disabled readers demonstrate some decoding problems. Nevertheless, the huge disparity between word recognition and comprehension skills development is a disturbing one.

Question 5 in Table 11-7 (see Appendix, p. 140) reports that visual and auditory modalities are used most often by reading teachers with only one-fourth of these reading teachers employing the kinesthetic modality.

If the results of this survey are at all accurate or even a crude estimation of the present status of an individual district's literacy programs, then the nation's schools are a long way from solving the illiteracy problem.

The solution to this situation appears to be very simple, at least in theory. No one discipline will ever solve the problem by itself. If all professionals concerned with the disabled reader were to pool their resources and talents—if they could stop guarding their frontiers and stop disallowing cross-over and learn to compromise and work together—then the illiteracy problem could possibly be solved.

REFERENCES

Basic Skills Agreement Preamble. U.S. Department of Education, Washington, D.C., 1979.

Harris, L. Harris Survey: Survival Literacy Study. Conducted for the National Reading Council, Washington, D.C.: Louis Harris and Associates, September, 1970.

International Literacy. Remarks of Ernest L. Boyer, United States Commissioner of Education at the International Literacy Day Conference, Washington, D.C. , 1978.

Memorandum of Understanding Between the United States Department of Health, Education, and Welfare, Office of Education, Right to Read Effort, and the United States Chamber of Commerce, Washington, D.C., 1979a.

Memorandum of Understanding Between the United States Department of Health, Education, and Welfare, Office of Education, Right to Read Effort, and the United States Department of the Navy, Washington, D.C., 1979b.

Navy Perspectives on a Joint Navy/Office of Education Literacy Training Program. Unpublished report, Washington, D.C., November 30, 1977.

Kilty, T. A study of the cultural complexity of our language. Unpublished report, U.S. Department of Education, Washington, D.C., 1978.

Rosners, S., Abrams, J., Daniels, P., & Schiffman, G. Focus on reading. *Journal of Learning Disabilities, 14* (8), 1981, p. 439.

Schiffman, G. Improving basic skills of Appalachian children. Unpublished Report to the Appalachian Regional Commission, Washington, D.C.: 1979a p. 9.

Schiffman, G. An intermin basic skills task force report. Unpublished report, U. S. Department of Education, Washington, D.C., 1979b.

Schiffman, G. Updating of reading disorders in the United States (1969 Working Paper). Unpublished Report, The John Hopkins University, Baltimore, Md., 1980.

Second Annual Report to Congress on the implementation of Public Law 94-142. Prepared by the Office of Special Education, U.S. Department of Education, Washington, D.C., 1980, p. 199.

APPENDIX

Table 11-1
Results of Questionnaire Concerning Literacy Programs
at the Local School Level*

Please respond *Yes* or *No* to the following questions according to your local school's reading program. (Not necessarily your personal convictions but *actually* what is happening now at the local site).

	Yes	No
a. All teachers (classroom, content & special) are involved in the teaching of reading.	42%	58%
b. There is conscious effort to identify pupils with reading disabilities early, i.e., K-1.	29%	71%
c. There is a teacher education program established for all personnel at local site.	25%	75%
d. There is community involvement in the actual instructional program, i.e., volunteers.	14%	86%
e. No one pedagogical procedure is recommended for all disabled readers.	87%	13%
f. The administration assumes leadership in establishing and coordinating the total reading program.	4%	96%
g. The school has established specific objectives and/or skills for the reading program.	31%	67%
h. Proper diagnostic tools have been obtained to ascertain where every pupil is in relation to above-mentioned objectives and/or skills.	11%	89%

National Response of 1,375 professional educators.

Table 11-2
Graduate Education of Interviewed Reading Teachers (N = 1375)

Grades	N	3 graduate courses or less in reading	4 graduate courses or more in reading (no graduate degree reading)	Graduate degree with major in reading	At least one graduate course Diagnosis of Learning Language		
					Reading Disabilities	Disabilities	Development or Speech
Elementary 1–6	895	2%	34%	64%	88%	5%	2%
Middle 5–8	169	4%	15%	81%	94%	8%	4%
Secondary 7–12	311	29%	30%	41%	43%	2%	0.6%
Total	1375	8%	31%	61%	78%	4%	2%

Table 11-3
Description of Reading Teacher's Major Responsibility (over 75% of time spent in activity)

Consultant and/or resource person for classroom teachers at local site	Diagnosis and/or reading instruction			Other activities
	Instructional groups (more than 7 pupils at one time)	Instructional groups (less than 7 pupils at one time)	Diagnosis and/or instruction in clinic or itinerate setting	
18%	24%	41%	7%	10%

Question 1. As a reading teacher who pays your salary?

Federal funds 21%   Nonfederal funds 79%

Question 2. As a reading teacher do you conduct teacher education programs?

Yes 19%   No 81%

If so, when?

Before school 8% After school 59% During school 25% Other 8%

Table 11-4
Descriptions of Pupils Serviced by Reading Teachers (over 75% of time spent in activity)*

All Pupils at local site	Achieving Pupils	Pupils with reading disabilities			All degrees of reading instruction	Other
		less than 2 years delayed in reading	more than 2 years delayed in reading			
17%	4%	23%	42%		10%	4%

*Elementary reading teachers only.

Table 11-5

Grade Level and Percentage of Pupils from Total School Population Assisted in Reading at Local Site (at least 75% of the time)

Group	Grade Level		Combination or Other	Percentage of Total School Population		
	Primary K-3	Intermediate 4–6		Less than 10%	11%–33%	Above 33%
Average percent of time of RT spent with group	35%	35%	30%	93%	7%	0%

Question 3. As a reading teacher do you instruct pupils with perceptual and/or motor deficits?

Yes 11% No 89%

Question 4. As a reading teacher are you involved in the diagnosis and/or instruction of special education children?

Yes 18% No 87%

If so, do you work alone or as a member of an interdisciplinary team?

Alone 70% Team member 30%

Table 11-6
Pedagogical Procedures Employed by Reading Teachers
(over 75% of time)

Procedure	% of Use
Basal	12%
Individualized	5%
Language Experience	3%
Programmed	6%
Eclectic	38%
Other Methods	36%

Table 11-7
Basic Skills Stressed by Reading Teacher (only check one)

Skill	Basic or Main Skill Stressed
Word Recognition	52%
Comprehension	19%
Study Skill	3%
Combination	26%
Other	0%

Question 5. What modalities do you employ in your remediation program?
(Check appropriate blanks)

Visual	Auditory	Kinesthetic	Tactile	Other
99%	88%	26%	53%	16%

12

The Evaluation and Instruction of the Severely Disabled Reader

One of the basic problems in evaluating disabled readers is defining the population. For example, there is no agreement on any one definition or on the name of the disablity with reading teachers using labels such as *remedial or disabled reader, strephosymbolia, associative learning disability, specific reading or language disability, congenital word blindness, primary reading retardation* and *developmental dyslexia*. One school district may refer to all disabled readers as *remedial;* in the same community another agency may use the term *remedial* for children with specific learning difficulties.

Additionally, most of the current definitions are expressed in terms of specific etiology or measurable performance. Historically, definitions cover genetic, organic, congenital, psychogenic, social, and educational causes and may include all students who are more than 2 years delayed in reading according to grade level or to only those children with "associative learning problems." However, no one has been able to clearly validate the 2 year cut-off, let alone agree on how to measure grade level achievement. The popular definition that defines the disabled reader as one who cannot learn to read by conventional techniques or conventional school organization is quite different from the definition that states that the disorder is totally organic in nature. In fact, another semantic "hangup" has developed since professionals have never been able to agree on a definition for the word "conventional."

Finally one has to recognize that, of all the handicapping categories, the field of learning disabilities (with a heavy focus on severe reading disabilities) has experienced a period of growth unparalleled by almost any other specialized field. Although the subject was virtually unheard of 25 years ago, modern education, psychology, and medicine have all contributed to its growing body of literature.

It is apparent that the accepted definition of learning disabilities first formulated by the National Advisory Committee on Dyslexia (1969) has its limitations, as the definition was one primarily of exclusion.

As late as the Fall of 1981, the representatives of the six organizations that constitute the National Joint Committee for Learning Disabilities (Hammill et al., 1981) reached unanimous agreement on a new definition of learning disabilities:

> Learning disabilities is a generic term that refers to a heterogeneous group of disorders manifested by significant difficulties in the acquisition and use of listening, speaking, reading, writing, reasoning or mathematical abilities. These disorders are intrinsic to the individual and presumed to be due to central nervous system dysfunction. Even though a learning disability may occur concomitantly with other handicapping conditions (e.g., sensory impairment, mental retardation, social and emotional disturbance) or environmental influences (e.g., cultural differences, insufficient/inappropriate instruction, psychogenic factors), it is not the direct result of those conditions or influences.

Nevertheless, most professionals agree that a learning disability is defined essentially in terms of an organic and neurological dysfunction of the cerebral processes. The purpose of any learning disabilities test battery is therefore to determine whether or not a minimal neurological dysfunction is impeding the child's ability to learn under otherwise normal conditions.

Unfortunately, there is still no agreement on what constitutes an appropriate diagnostic battery. Different districts continue to use different criteria and diagnostic tools in identifying the learning disabled child. This "individualization" results in major differences in "child finds." For example, the Bureau of Education for the Handicapped (1979) (now Office of Special Education) reported to Congress that out of the 570,142 potentially learning disabled children not identified during the 1977–1978 school years, Texas overidentified 27,041 and New York failed to identify 95,506.

Because of this lack of agreement, we cannot even guess at the number of learning disabled children. Experts quote figures from one-half of one percent to 20 percent of the total school population.

ADMINISTRATIVE AND EDUCATIONAL INERTIA

Administrators often do not understand that there are a large number of children who have not been successful learners with traditional methods. Too often, lip service has been given to the "individual" child, "individualization" of programs, etc., but in reality children are exposed to traditional mass instruction.

An effective program may take years to be proven successful. If administrators are not completely sold on the program, they may fear that they are doing something just too unorthodox and expensive. Pressure from school board members and the public can build rapidly, and the tendency to look for the speedy magic panacea can become overwhelming.

The real problem may be that the decision making personnel are often too far removed from the classroom to observe the failures and to search for newer ideas about the causes. In large school districts, ideas must be forced through a great number of committees in order to gain acceptance. The danger of dilution and modification of these ideas after exposure to the committees is, therefore, a serious factor. It is difficult for anyone removed from a day-to-day contact with children to be highly motivated about the small ideas and creative approaches that actually help children learn.

A major problem is the lack of knowledge and understanding on the part of administrators. Innovation is hard for many experienced educators, and inertia will inhibit experimentation and the development of new programs. Unfortunately, no effective program can be developed without administrative approval and leadership.

ORGANIZATION OF THE REMEDIATION PROGRAM

Once the school system has defined a population of disabled readers and the educators have agreed on a basic philosophy for implementation, then the next stage is the actual organization and administration of the remediation program.

Structure of the Remediation Program

A decision must be made on what type of organizational program should be provided (e.g., assistance in the regular classroom, remediation in small groups, involvement in a one to one tutoring program, or attendance in a self-contained special education class or in a full-time school or clinic). Frequently, different departments (such as general instruction versus special education) develop conflicts that can retard the growth and development of the program. The prevalent attitude among many concerned but semi-informed educators is that the disabled child is so special that he or she must receive a special placement, thereby implying the necessity of his or her removal from even a modified program of studies. Unfortunately, with this philosophy in mind, a child labeled "disabled" may sit in a regular classroom waiting for special help or special education placement. Some classroom teachers become so terrified by the diagnosis that they avoid contact with the disabled reader. If the educators become too fearful and concerned, the hopelessness they feel in trying to help may result in their "standing still" until they can afford to establish a clinic. Although reduced class size, individual instruction, or an interdisciplinary clinic are undoubtedly ideal, the remedial reader's situation can be greatly helped within the regular classroom structure with appropriate techniques.

A basic premise of remedial teaching is that each child needs to work at his or her own developmental level. This level may be different for each area of learning. When grouping children, their levels of education and social development must also be taken into account. If the only factors considered when children are grouped are those of decoding, speed and comprehension, then it will be difficult to see any real change in the teaching approach. The top group does what the bottom group does—only faster. Where does this leave the child with excellent comprehension but faulty decoding ability? Where does this leave the child with both faulty comprehension and decoding? Unfortunately, it usually leaves the child in the *same* reading group, using the *same* techniques as the top group—only moving slower.

Evaluation Procedures

As the learning disability field has grown, so too has its criticism. Many learning disability specialists admit that the field has been rife with ambiguities and contradictions from its inception, and thus they recognize the need for less confusion and greater clarity. In addition, recent publications have raised sobering questions about prescribed diagnostic and therapeutic guidelines.

The haphazard and controversial approach to the solution of a child's learning problems has to be replaced with a reliable, coordinate, effective, and economically feasible method of systematic early identification and diagnosis. This explains why the Education of All Handicapped Children Act, Public Law 94-142, calls for a multidisciplinary team to make the proper evaluation. The child has to be assessed in all areas related to the learning disability, including, where appropriate, health, vision, hearing, social and emotional status, general intelligence, academic performance, communicative status, and motor abilities. The academic areas to be assessed include:

1. Oral expression
2. Listening comprehension
3. Written expression
4. Basic reading skills
5. Reading comprehension
6. Mathematics calculation
7. Mathematics reasoning

If the team finds that a student has a severe discrepancy between achievement and intellectual ability in one of these areas and if this discrepancy is not the result of a visual, hearing or motor handicap, mental retardation, emotional disturbance, environmental, cultural, or economic disadvantage, then the student can be identified as having a specific learning disability.

As mentioned earlier, because of the vagueness of the definition, districts interpret "severe discrepancy" in various ways. Unfortunately, most objective measures (i.e., formulae), have also proven unreliable and invalid.

The Maryland Learning Disabilities Project (1982) (Table 12-1) is currently assessing and reassessing a "case study" evaluation approach. In this project all of the professionals who have evaluated a student meet together in an interdisciplinary approach, discuss their findings, and together conclude whether or not, and to what extent, the student needs "special" education to remediate his or her disability. It was initially concluded that the multidisciplinary team should have the following documentation:

1. Individual standardized educational assessment in the areas of language arts, spelling, reading, mathematics, and writing
2. Educational assessments to be performed by personnel within the education discipline (classroom teachers, administrators, resource teachers, reading specialists, special education teachers, and Title I teachers)
3. Description of cognitive functioning and written validated data certifying average intelligence and learning disability
4. Cognitive functioning determination to be made by personnel from the disciplines of psychology and speech pathology*

This interdisciplinary approach makes good sense and is applicable for all diagnoses, whether they are special education, reading disabilities, Title I, basic skills, or general education. Of course, the special education diagnosis, because of legal implications, has to follow a more formal procedure. The multidisciplinary meeting is usually called an ARD (annual review and dismissal) and the remediation plan is an IEP (individualized educational plan).

One purpose of a multidisciplinary approach to diagnosing a learning disability is to compensate for the weaknesses in diagnosis that results from relying on one person's assessment. The need to look at all data sources, objective and subjective, and to use the clinical sensitivities of the team members seems crucial. Evaluators must not fall into the trap of being overly concerned with a numerical "severe discrepancy." Furthermore, the team must strive to validate all of its "measures" of underlying psychological processes through comparisons of assessments, behaviors, observation, development and history, making sure that they don't handicap the child when poor teaching or other environmental factors have caused the problem.

Richard Mainzer, Chairman of the Maryland Learning Disabilities Project, states that a recently developed student profile sheet appears to assist educators in organizing child data in a nonmetric clinical approach that aids the interdisciplinary team in their evaluation and instructional design.

This student profile is used during screening, assessment, and evaluation. It is especially useful in organizing the disparate pieces of information from the diverse disciplines. Individual assessments

---

*assessments limited to linguistic function

considered separately can lead to a fragmentary picture of the whole child and to fragmentary plans for instruction. Table 12-1 demonstrates the Maryland Learning Disabilities Project Student Profile. The various assessment factors are arranged across the top of the form.

The first group (Section A) contains those factors which may cause underachievement in nonlearning disabled students. The second group (Section B) represents the seven areas of achievement described in federal regulations. It is these seven areas that are specifically compared to the student's educational aptitude in determining the existence of "severe discrepancy." The final group (Section C) is made up of factors that may contribute to or effect a severe discrepancy in learning disabled students.

If the team decides there is a severe discrepancy then the team will look at Section A and Section C. If the team decides the severe discrepancy is primarily caused by any of the factors or combination of factors in Section A, then the child is not learning disabled. On the other hand, if the team decides that one or more of the factors in Section C are the primary cause of the severe discrepancy, then the child is learning disabled.

Dr. Marjorie Johnson (1975) explains why a multidisciplinary evaluation is so necessary for all severe reading disabilities. She reminds the reader that there may be many reasons why a child has not been able to profit from an instructional program through which others have learned to read. The factors that interfere with the functioning of the individual's intelligence for purposes of acquiring reading skills and abilities are varied. The influence of the following factors has been widely investigated: visual functioning, auditory functioning, speech and language development, reversal tendency, memory span, associative learning ability, and social and emotional adjustment. In any particular case, some or all of these factors, and others less widely investigated, have an inhibitive effect on the acquisition of reading ability.

Pedagogical Procedures

Once the reading disabled child is identified and placed in the appropriate program, the teachers must provide the proper pedagogical techniques. Regretfully, popular reading techniques are not easily changed.

Table 12-1

Maryland Learning Disabilities Project: Student Profile

N. No Problem Indicated
P. Problem Indicated

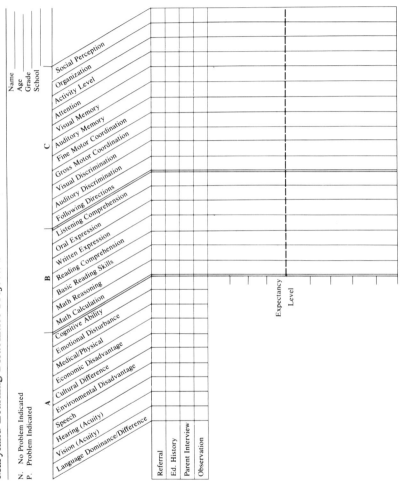

148

When a specific learning problem can be defined, individualized teaching methods, materials, and techniques should be utilized by the school system to help these children to circumvent or to overcome their particular learning disability.

Unfortunately, in some programs every remedial pupil is exposed to one particular technique. The selection of the specific pedagogical procedure may depend to a large extent on the training of the clinician and on the bias of the diagnostic center. Educators embrace the philosophy of individual differences, but too often accept the "one right way" of teaching reading to all disabled readers. Pupils and teachers alike have had to adjust to the one procedure instead of the teacher and technique adjusting to the needs of the child. Too often teachers have followed one policy blindly because some authority has said, "This is the way." Experience has demonstrated the fact that there is no magic panacea for all children. These severely disabled have one consistent syndrome, besides their disability, and that is inconsistency. The clinician must select the appropriate technique through diagnostic teaching and use all sensory pathways to reinforce the weak memory patterns. The method or combination of methods that helps the child is the right method. A teacher must have considerable training and proficiency in all pedagogical procedures to follow this eclectic approach.

The Maryland Learning Disabilities Project has concluded that the general goals and objectives of programming for learning disabled students are the same as for all other students. In addition, there are special goals related to the unique learning needs of each child. Based on this philosophy, the following is proposed as a model for instructional programming for learning disabled students. The four components, or instructional strategies, are (1) modified developmental teaching, (2) remedial teaching, (3) adaptive teaching, and (4) instruction in functional life skills.

Modified Developmental Teaching, as built into the regular methods and content of instruction of the school, is used with the learning disabled student to achieve those goals of education established for all students. Developmental teaching is defined as those materials, methods, and management techniques approved by the local educational agencies (LEA) that are usually successful with normally developing children. Necessary modifications to meet the unique needs of the learning disabled students may be provided.

Remediation Teaching is defined as those methods, materials, and management techniques selected to ameliorate a learning disabled child's specific areas of disability identified through the assessment process and stated in the individual education plan (IEP).

Adaptive Teaching is defined as those methods, materials, and management techniques selected to circumvent a learning disabled student's specific areas of disabilities and maximize areas of abilities. Adaptive teaching is synonymous with compensatory teaching (i.e., helping the student compensate for the disabilities).

Instruction in Functional Life Skills is defined as those methods, materials, and management techniques designed to teach appropriate social and adaptive behavior for a particular student's life situations.

Instructional strategies will vary with the level of service and severity of disability in the child. The emphasis of instructional strategies will also vary with the age and educational history of the child. With a very young child, emphasis may be developmental rather than remedial, since the young child may not have been exposed to appropriate instruction or may have developed inappropriate learning behaviors to the point where he or she is far enough behind to need remediation.

At the elementary level, major emphasis needs to be placed on modified developmental teaching and remedial teaching, with adaptive teaching when appropriate. For some secondary learning disabled students who have been exposed to remedial instruction without success, it may be appropriate to place greater emphasis on adaptive teaching, circumventing the disability rather than remediating it. Remedial teaching may be appropriate for others. If a student has received special education services for a long period of time, with limited success and consequent motivational problems, an adaptive program may be indicated. If, however, a student has received little or no remedial services, or is progressing well and continues to be motivated, a remedial program should be continued, supplemented by a strong developmental program modified when necessary to insure success for each student. Adaptive teaching in all content and skill areas needs to be built into all levels of programming in order to insure ongoing success in the regular classroom.

Instruction in functional life skills is vital for some learning disabled students at all levels in order to help students master the developmental tasks appropriate for their present and future life situations. For some students, this may involve classroom behavior, social interactions with peers and adults, social perception and self-perception, and emotional adjustment. For others, it may include prevocational and vocational preparation or training of survival skills.

Since the goal of the learning disabilities program is to provide an integrated program, incorporating both the regular class and the special class, the need for open two-way communication among all staff members involved in serving the student is critical. Due to the numbers of staff who may be involved in serving the needs of the learning disabled student, it is essential that one person be designated as the case manager. The case manager, as designated by the admission review and dismissal (ARD) committee, will be responsible for facilitating the implementation of services and time lines of the individualized evaluation program (IEP). The role of advocacy and personal involvement in each child's progress will be the primary responsibility of this case manager.

The "average" child acquires adequate reading ability through visual and auditory clues with no kinesthetic stimulation except that involved in speech and in subsequent writing. Regardless of how much improved the program of instruction in reading is for him, some few very capable children will still not succeed. These are the people who, for a variety of reasons, have unusual difficulty in forming associations between experience and printed symbols. Even when these students are exposed to a program of instruction through which people of similar mental age learn to read well, they may remain completely unable to look at a printed word or group of words and connect meaning with them. These individuals are given different labels depending on the training and bias of the clinician. Very often medical professionals call them "dyslexic," reading specialists label them "disabled or clinically or associatively learning disabled," and special educators give them the diagnosis of "specific learning disabled."

For those individuals with this disability, special methods are necessary. They are able, however, to develop good reading abilities. To do this, they must use for word learning techniques that allow them to use tactile and/or kinesthetic clues as well as visual and auditory clues. *VAKT,* as this technique is called, involves visual, auditory, kinesthetic and tactile stimulation in the learning process. Visual stimulation is that which the individual receives through the eye; auditory stimulation is that received through the ear; kinesthetic stimulation is that which arises in the musculature, in the tendons, and so on, as the result of body movements or tensions within the body; tactile stimulation is that which arises in the skin from contact with outside objects.

The use of kinesthetic and tactile methods has been in evidence virtually as long as have organized programs of education. Greek and Roman writings give accounts of guiding the child's hand over a written model or providing boards on which the outlines of letters were cut into deep grooves for tracing.

Two special pedagogical techniques, the Fernald and the Gillingham, are often considered in the remediation of these severely disabled readers. Both approaches involve the use of as many kinds of stimulation as necessary for acquiring and retaining the ability to recognize words.

Table 12-2 details some of the approaches employed in reading instruction. The list does not include all techniques nor does it suggest that these approaches exist in isolation. However, it is imperative that all of the professionals involved in a child's reading instructional program agree on techniques that are compatible. For

Table 12-2
Methods of Reading Instruction

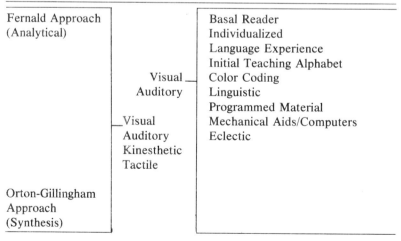

Fernald Approach (Analytical)	Visual Auditory	Basal Reader
		Individualized
		Language Experience
		Initial Teaching Alphabet
		Color Coding
		Linguistic
		Programmed Material
	Visual Auditory Kinesthetic Tactile	Mechanical Aids/Computers
		Eclectic
Orton-Gillingham Approach (Synthesis)		

example, it would not be beneficial for any student to receive reading remediation in the Fernald and Gillingham approaches at the same period of time.

This method employs a series of graded readers with a controlled vocabulary. It is usually used in a teacher−directed reading activity spelled out in an accompanying manual.

Individualized Reading Approach

In this approach students read independently (often in trade books) and are instructed individually by the teacher in relation to the book being read and then in small groups for skill development. Any method by which students are allowed to progress independently of the group is usually termed "individualized."

Language Experience Approach

This approach has students discuss a common experience and then dictate or write a short story about it. The story then becomes the material used for teaching reading, including the mastery of a basic sight vocabulary.

In some clinical situations this approach, coupled with the Fernald multisensory technique, has proven effective with disabled readers.

Initial Teaching Alphabet Approach

This is one of several systems devised to attack the problem that any number of phonemes in the English language may have several ways of being represented by the English system of orthography. Initial Teaching Alphabet's (ITA's) proposed solution is to make a *temporary change* in the orthography of the English language for beginning readers through the creation of a very consistent phoneme-grapheme relationship.

Color Coding Approach

Color coding is another approach to solving the problem of the inconsistent orthography of the English language. It superimposes consistency upon standing English orthography by adding the dimension of color. The color coders superimpose a single, invariant color upon a given vowel sound in the printing of their materials regardless of the variety of ways in which that sound is normally represented in written form.

Linguistics Approach

The solution proposed by the present day descriptive linguists to the inconsistent orthography of the English language is one of delay. In brief, they advocate the presentation of words that only represent regular or consistent relationships between sounds and printed symbols in the beginning stages of reading. This is followed by a delayed, gradual, and systematic introduction of irregular phoneme-grapheme correspondences.

Programmed Material Approach

In this approach there is a sequential presentation of bits of information in small steps or frames, each requiring a response on the part of the student. Answers are then revealed for immediate feedback. Students progress at their own rate, the teacher's role is to monitor progress and administer progress tests at specified intervals. Linguistically oriented material that stresses phoneme-grapheme correspondences is usually used for reading programs.

Mechanical Aids and Computers Approach

The application of mechanical and electronic technology to aid the teaching of the communication skills has gained great support, enthusiasm, and anticipation in the education community. Tachistoscopes and pacers have been widely used in speed reading programs. Presently, some schools use personal computers to help students with specific subjects, such as mathematics or reading, and to challenge high achievers; nowhere are the benefits of learning with personal computers more dramatic than with the handicapped. There is no question that the surface has barely been scratched in the educational and therapeutic use of technology for all children.

Eclectic Approach

This is the smorgasbord technique. The student is exposed to a combination of approaches and/or methods of reading instruction. This does not have to be classified as a "hit or miss" procedure. A skilled teacher using an effective diagnostic–prescriptive approach may effectively employ this technique.

Fernald Approach

Teachers employing the Fernald approach usually begin with a tracing step. At this stage learners listen as the teacher writes the word. The learners observe the writing, say the word as they trace (continuing until they can write the word), and say it as they write it. As they progress, they no longer need the tracing, but otherwise follow the same type of procedure. Throughout the stages, words are learned as wholes, being pronounced naturally and in syllables as they are traced, studied, or written. This tracing technique is an attempt to achieve maximum stimulation for word learning.

Gillingham Approach

In contrast to the Fernald analytical approach, the Gillingham is a synthesis procedure. The Gillingham technique advocates teaching the sounds of the letters and then building these letter sounds into words, like bricks into a wall. Many educators associate this method with the familiar "phonetic" or "sound" technique. The difference lies in the fact that the Gillingham approach is based on the close association of visual, auditory, and kinesthetic elements.

Historically, and from a realistic point of view, most disability programs have focused on teaching the reading disabled child how to "break the word recognition code." In other words, remediation emphasis is on basic reading skills, not comprehension.

Two events may soon turn the emphasis completely around. One event involves recent national assessments indicating that students are still having difficulty with comprehension. Reading specialists are becoming more competent in the area of critical thinking and comprehension and are focusing increasingly on that area. The second event is that *reading comprehension* is considered one of the seven achievement areas considered in Public Law 94-142's learning disability category. Unfortunately, professionals still know very little about this area. Comprehension skills are varied in type and depth.

The variation of demands in comprehension are clearly demonstrated in an informal reading inventory used at Temple University. The third reader level selection tells the reader that a dog should have one meal in summer and two in winter. To check factual recall the teacher may ask, "How many meals a day should you give a dog in summer?" Unfortunately, this is a very common type of question. How much more enlightening is the question from the informal reading inventory, "How many meals a day should you give a dog in July?" Too frequently the answer is "It didn't say" or "July wasn't even in the story." The second question taps a child's ability to do inferential thinking—to manipulate the facts so that a higher level of understanding arises.

Any good comprehension check should not only check straight factual recall but deeper, critical thinking skills. Many authorities believe such measures should be roughly 50 percent vocabulary which really cuts across both the factual and the critical areas. However, because of the trend toward verbalism, more weight on critical reading seems appropriate.

In reviewing a lesson of about 145 words written at the high third or fourth grade readability level, we can check some of the different types of critical comprehension that can be evaluated.

Strong Bow rode into the valley. The sun, directly overhead, beat down with increasing fury. The Black Toe chief was very tired. The raid had not been successful. One third of his men had been killed. Six mounted braves trailed close behind their chief. Small puffs of dust arose from the horses' hooves, and their manes lay motionless against their wet sides. The chief was very sad. He was returning to his village in disgrace. He had no booty; he had no scalps. Slowly the small band headed home towards the mountains. As the sun sank behind the mountain range, they were still far from their loved ones. The chief decided to stop for the night. The men needed rest. In fact, this would be the final resting place for some of the unlucky warriors.

The description of the skills evaluated by the comprehension check are as follows (description numbers correspond to comprehension question numbers):

1. *Semantic variation* of vocabulary tests and reader's ability to identify a similar usage of a given word from the selection.
2. *Main idea* tests the ability to identify the key or most important idea in the story.
3. *Generalization* tests the ability to form a general conclusion of principle applicable to an entire class of data on the basis of a limited number of specific instances stated in a selection.
4. *Association of ideas* tests the ability to see the relationship among ideas in a series.
5. *Antecedent* tests the ability to recognize the word or words to which a selected pronoun refers.
6. *Analogy* tests the ability to perceive relationship between two pairs of ideas.
7. *Sequence* tests the ability to determine a time sequence.
8. *Extraneous ideas* tests the ability to determine relevancy of ideas to a selection.

9–13.   *Inference* tests the ability to draw a specific conclusion from facts explicitly stated.

CRITICAL COMPREHENSION EXERCISE

1. The sentence which uses the word *range* just as it is used in the story is:
    a)   The band of Indians ranged over the country
    b)   The cook made the breakfast on the range
    c)   The gunners adjust the range of the cannon
    d)   The climbers reached the top of the highest range
    e)   The boys went to the shooting range
2. The main idea in the story is that:
    a)   Strong Bow was very tired
    b)   The Indians were returning home after an unsuccessful raid
    c)   The Indians had no booty or scalps
    d)   One-third of the Indians had been killed
    e)   The Indians were still far from their families at the end of the day
3. From the story we should not believe that all of the Indians . . .
    a)   rode horses
    b)   were Black Toes
    c)   were tired
    d)   returned home in disgrace
    e)   returned home safely
4. The row with ideas from the story that belong together is . . .
    a)   Strong Bow, chief, dust
    b)   booty, scalps, sun
    c)   names, hooves, sides
    d)   home, families, hooves
    e)   puffs, dust, manes
5. In the sentence, "As the sun sank behind the mountain range they were still far from their loves ones," the word *their* stands for . . .
    a)   horses'
    b)   Strong Bow's
    c)   Indian's

    d) Black Toe's Tribe's

    e) Indians'

6. Strong Bow is to Black Toe's Tribe as _____ is to the United States of America.

7. The first sentence out of order is:

    a) The Indians rode into the valley.

    b) The chief decided to stop for the night.

    c) The June sun was very hot.

    d) Small puffs of dust arose from the horses' hooves.

    e) The band of Indians headed towards the mountain.

8. The idea not found in the story is that:

    a) Six of the horses had been killed

    b) The raiders needed rest

    c) The Indians were far away from their homes

    d) The Indians were travelling towards the west

    e) The band of Indians would lose some more men before they returned home

9. What time of the day was it when the Indians rode into the valley?

10. Was it a wet or dry country? How do you know?

11. Was it a calm or windy day? How do you know?

12. How many Indians started out on this raid?

13. In what direction was the band headed?

Development of this type of comprehension, of course, is not only in the hands of the reading or learning disability specialist. All teachers have a responsibility to check comprehension and to develop comprehension skills, utilizing the critical reading area. There is no question that this type of comprehension lends itself very easily to social studies and science material. There is no question, also, that this is just a small sampling of the different kinds of critical comprehension that can be developed. When one looks at all of this, one realizes the tremendous responsibility that is placed upon the educator: developing good word recognition skills and good comprehension skills in the proper proportion; looking warily at all of the biased groups; questioning all of the magic panaceas and cure-alls; keeping in mind the different types of comprehension; and still seeing the ultimate goal—that the student should read for meaning, for enjoyment, and for learning regardless of the disability.

REFERENCES

Bureau of Education for the Handicapped. Progress toward a free appropriate public education. Unpublished report prepared for U.S. Department of Health, Education, and Welfare. Washington, D.C., 1979, p. 163.

Daniels, P., & Schiffman, G. Watch out for the swinging pendulum. *The Australian Journal of the Education of Backward Children, 13:*1, 1966, 3–8.

Dwyer, K., Mainzer, R., Mowery, F., Mitchell, D., Rofel, M., & Simon, K. The Maryland learning disability project. Unpublished report. Baltimore, MD: Maryland State Department of Education, 1982, p. 17.

Hammill, D., Leigh, J., McNutt, G., & Larsen, S. A new definition of learning disabilities. *Learning Disability Quarterly.* Fall, 1981, p. 336–341.

Informal Reading Inventory. Diagnostic Division, The Reading Clinic, Department of Psychology, Temple University, Philadelphia, PA., (undated).

Johnson, M. The Fernald approach. Unpublished paper. Temple University, Philadelphia, PA., 1975.

National Advisory Committee on Dyslexia. Reading disorders in the United States. Unpublished report prepared for U.S. Department of Health, Education, and Welfare, Washington, D.C., 1969.

ANSWER KEY TO CRITICAL COMPREHENSION EXERCISE

1. (d)
2. (b)
3. (e)
4. (c)
5. (e)
6. Ronald Reagan (or current President)
7. (b)
8. (a)
9. Noon (sun directly overhead)
10. Dry (small puffs of dust)
11. Calm (manes lay motionless)
12. 10 (nine braves plus the chief)
13. West (band headed towards the mountain; sun sank behind the mountain range)

13

Legal Considerations for the Handicapped

THE SYSTEMS OF LAW

At the three levels of government—federal, state and local—there are four sources of law. These include: constitutions (charters at the local levels), statutes (ordinances at the local level), court decisions, and administrative regulations.

Statutes and ordinances are laws passed by legislatures. Thus, federal statutes are passed by the U. S. Congress, the Senate, and the House of Representatives and are the laws of the United States. They supersede inconsistent state and local laws and any conflicting regulations. Statutes generally include a statement of purpose. For example, Public Law 94-142 reads, "It is the purpose of this act to assure that all handicapped children have available to them. . . ." It is important to mention that while statutes are more specific than constitutional provisions, they are rarely self-explanatory or self-enforcing.

Administrative Regulations

Legislatures sometimes authorize administrative agencies to develop specific regulations to enforce a statute. While these regulations usually carry the power of law, they may be challenged legally as exceeding the authority granted to the agency by the legislature.

160

Federal Regulations are developed by a notice and/or comment rule-making procedure. The agency drafts a proposed regulation and publishes it in the *Federal Register* with a deadline for receipt of public comments. For some regulations public hearings may be held in which the agency ultimately involved revises the proposed rules and circulates a second version for additional review and comment. Final regulations are published in the *Federal Register* and in the *Code of Federal Regulations*.

Court Decisions

Court decisions are judicial interpretations of constitutional provisions, statutes, and regulations. The federal judicial system includes three levels of courts: U.S. District Courts, U.S. Circuit Courts, and the U.S. Supreme Court. There are 93 federal district courts serving all or part of the 50 states, the District of Columbia, the Virgin Islands, Puerto Rico, the Canal Zone, and Guam. Federal circuit courts hear appeals of district court rulings as well as certain special types of cases.

State courts normally hear only cases involving state constitutional law, statutes and administrative regulations, as well as contract or tort cases. They are also empowered to hear and decide federal constitutional and civil rights cases. An example of this would be a suit brought under Section 504 of the Rehabilitation Act of 1973, (PL 93-112).

Parallel to federal district courts are state trial-level courts known variously as superior courts or courts of general jurisdiction. Larger states have two levels of appeals courts, generally referred to as the state court of appeals and the state supreme court. Cities or countries normally have their own courts whose jurisdiction is limited to matters of local law and whose decisions can be appealed to the state trial courts.

LAWS AND THE HANDICAPPED

Laws that govern services for learning disabled and other handicapped children have dramatically changed over the last decade. While the Fourteenth Amendment guarantees equal protection under the law to all people, this has not always been enforced.

Under the Constitution, any state in the country that provides a public education to its children is required to do so regardless of that child's handicap. Theoretically the Constitution provides free and appropriate programs to all individuals, but there are many instances in which the law is not implemented or there are significant efforts to support noncompliance. It was not until the 1970s that children with learning disabilities were accorded their basic rights.

Historically, individuals who were severely handicapped were commonly excluded from public school programs on the basis that they could not benefit from the education. It was not until 1954 in the U.S. Supreme Court in the Brown *vs* The Board of Education (347 U.S. 483) that it was decided that *any* child could benefit from education. State laws that allowed and encouraged exclusion to this ruling began to be challenged in federal court. Two landmark federal cases have had a profound effect on the rights of the handicapped. Both of these landmark cases maintain the basic constitutional assumption that handicapped children are also entitled to equal protection of the laws and may not be treated differently without due process. The first case involved the Pennsylvania Association for Retarded Children *vs* The Commonwealth of Pennsylvania (334F. Supp. 1257 E.D. Pa. 1971). This specific decision resulted in the determination that the State of Pennsylvania owed retarded children an appropriate program of education and training. The second landmark case involved the District of Columbia in Mills *vs* The Board of Education. In this case, a similar decision was rendered with the major exception being that the guarantee of the right to education was applied to children with all types of handicaps. Specifically noted were those children who had been labeled as behavioral problems, emotionally disturbed, and/or hyperactive.

The impetus created by these two landmark cases resulted in a massive number of law suits and class actions against local boards of education (LEAs). Immediately following the Mills decision, 36 right-to-education decisions followed in 27 different states. Educators, parents, and other professionals quickly realized that it was time to establish some type of a federal standard that would assure that handicapped children could be provided and guaranteed equal protection under the law as outlined in the Fourteenth Amendment.

It should be noted that in 1966 Congress created a Bureau of Education for the Handicapped specifically to address the existing and anticipated problems of integrating severely handicapped children into public schools. Following the Pennsylvania and District of Columbia decisions, a bill was introduced into the Senate to expand the federal role. Many of these provisions were reflected in Public Law 93-380 of 1974.

Section 504

While the Constitution provides many rights for the people, it has been historically obvious that the handicapped were discriminated against not only in school-related matters but also in areas concerning civil rights. In 1971 the United States Senate began an effort that was to result in an amendment to the Civil Rights Act. Advocates for the handicapped insisted that handicapped citizens' civil rights were being violated. Legislation was enacted and Section 504 was included in the final section of the Vocational Rehabilitation Act of 1973. Section 504 provided that no handicapped person may be "excluded from, denied the benefit of, or be subjected to discrimination because of his or her handicap by any program which received federal funds." The signing of these final regulations was significant in that it required dramatic changes in the actions and attitudes of agencies, institutions, and individuals who had been receiving federal funds. Final regulations for Section 504 were published in May of 1977, and these specific provisions are supposed to be closely monitored in an agency receiving federal support.

Public Law 94-103

Federal courts also quickly began to recognize that many handicapped individuals were inappropriately placed in residential institutions and that, once there, little was done to return them to a more "normalized" setting. The Developmentally Disabled Act was, therefore, amended in 1975 to include a Bill of Rights section, whose specific purpose was to specify the rights of the developmentally disabled persons.

The final regulations for Public Law 94-103, the Developmentally Disabled Assistance and Bill of Rights Act, were published in January of 1977. This specific act placed certain requirements on state departments of education to assure appropriateness of placement, to provide interaction between residential and community facilities, and to provide for the educational need of all of its handicapped people.

Public Law 94-142

In 1975 Congress passed the Education for All Handicapped Children Act (PL 94-142).* This law went into effect in September of 1978 and made it possible for states and localities to receive funds to assist in the education of handicapped children. It is important to note, however, that the definition of handicapped children in specific categories continues to plague the educational profession. Many of the definitions are so global that they tend to confuse those individuals who are trying to develop appropriate programs.

The following definitions of handicapped children have been extracted from Public Law 94-142, which assures:

> . . . that all handicapped children have available to them . . . a free appropriate public education which emphasizes special education and related services designed to meet their unique needs, to assure that the rights of handicapped children and their parents or guardians are protected, to assist States and localities to provide for the education of all handicapped children, and to assess and assure the effectiveness of efforts to educate handicapped children (PL 94-142).

"Handicapped children" means those children who have been determined through appropriate assessment to have temporary or long-term special educational needs arising from cognitive, emotional, physical factors, or any combination of these factors. Their ability to meet general educational objectives is impaired to a degree whereby the services available in the general education program are inadequate in preparing them to achieve their educational potential.

"Handicapped children" includes those children who have been considered:

1. *Deaf,* which describes a hearing impairment that is so severe that the child is impaired in processing linguistic information through hearing, with or without amplification, which adversely affects educational performance.
2. *Deaf-blind,* which describes concomitant hearing and visual impairments, the combination of which causes such severe communication and other developmental and educational prob-

---

*Congressional efforts are currently underway to significantly reduce many of the provisions mandated under PL 94-142. The reader is encouraged to monitor the progress of these efforts.

lems that the children cannot be accommodated in special education programs solely for deaf or blind children.

3. *Hard of hearing,* which describes a hearing impairment, whether permanent or fluctuating, which adversely affects a child's educational performance but which is not included under the definition of "deaf" in this section.

4. *Mentally retarded,* which describes significantly subaverage general intellectual functioning existing concurrently with deficits in adaptive behavior and manifested during the developmental period, which adversely affects a child's educational performance.

5. *Multi-handicapped,* which describes concomitant impairments (such as mentally retarded-blind, mentally retarded-orthopedically impaired, etc.), the combination of which causes such severe educational problems that the children cannot be accommodated in special education programs solely for one of the impairments. The term does not include deaf-blind children.

6. *Orthopedically impaired,* which descibes a severe orthopedic impairment which adversely affects a child's educational performance. The term include impairments causes by congenital anomalies (for example, club foot, absence of some member, etc.), impairments caused by disease (for example, poliomyelitis, bone tuberculosis, etc.), and impairments from other causes (for example, cerebral palsy, amputations, and fractures or burns, which cause contractures).

7. *Other health impaired,* which describes limited strength, vitality, or alertness, due to chronic or acute health problems (such as heart condition, tuberculosis, rheumatic fever, nephritis, asthma, sickle cell anemia, hemophilia, epilepsy, lead poisoning, leukemia, or diabetes), which adversely affects a child's educational performance.

8. Seriously emotionally disturbed, which describes a condition in which one or more of the following characteristics is exhibited over a long period of time, adversely affecting educational performance to a marked degree:

   A. An inability to learn which cannot be explained by intellectual, sensory, or health factors
   B. An inability to build or maintain satisfactory interpersonal relationships with peers and teachers

    C. Inappropriate types of behavior or feelings under normal circumstances

    D. A general pervasive mood of unhappiness or depression

    E. A tendency to develop physical symptoms or fears associated with personal or school problems

The term includes children who are schizophrenic or autistics. The term does *not* include children who are socially maladjusted, unless they are seriously emotionally disturbed.

9. *Speech impaired,* which describes a communication disorder, such as stuttering, impaired articulation, a language impairment, or a voice impairment, which adversely affects a child's educational performance.

10. *Visually handicapped,* which describes a visual impairment which, even with correction, adversely affects a child's educational performance. The term includes both partially seeing and blind children.

11. *Learning disability,* which, as defined in the regulations for Public Law 94-142, means:

> A disorder in one or more of the basic psychological processes involved in understanding or in using language, spoken or written, which may manifest itself in imperfect ability to listen, think, speak, read, write, spell, or to do mathematical calculations. The term includes such conditions as perceptual handicaps, brain injury, minimal brain dysfunction, dyslexia, and development aphasia. The term does not include children who have learning problems which are primarily the result of visual, hearing, or motor handicaps, or mental retardation, or of environmental, cultural or economic disadvantage (PL 94-142, 121a. 5[9]).

Family Education Rights and Privacy Act

The Family Education Rights and Privacy Act (FERPA), more commonly referred to as the Buckley Amendment, was passed in 1974 (see Chapter 14). It provided handicapped children and their parents with the right to know all information and to challenge or correct any errors in the school record. In addition, it provided parents with the right to control the accessibility of their child's school record.

Today the courts and state legislators, supported by recent

strong federal laws, have made it reasonable to assume that a handicapped child can receive an education. The decades when schools were permitted to exclude certain groups of children and to declare that some were not capable of being educated because of their disabilities are hopefully past. Laws do not enforce themselves, however. It will take a conscious and concerted effort to make sure that the safeguards inherent in the laws are rigorously applied.

One of the most important results of recent federal legislation is the specific requirement for state education and developmental disability agencies to develop statewide plans for administering services for the handicapped. These plans require assurance that all federal requirements are being met, and, before any federal funding can go to a state, the plan must be in existence and approved. Those individuals interested in the legal aspects of working with handicapped individuals, and specifically the learning disabled, should carefully review their state plan for assurance that safeguards as well as guarantees under the Constitution and public laws are being met.

Concept of Restrictiveness

The passage of Public Law 94-142 provides surface legislative assurances of fair treatment to handicapped students. By this law, the handicapped individual must receive a free and appropriate education. While there has been little discussion concerning the definition of the term "free" in the law, there has been much discussion and confusion over the term "appropriate." The word *appropriate* extends the implications of the law beyond the issues of equal rights. It has yet to be operationally defined and, unfortunately, continues to be defined both narrowly and globally, depending upon the state in which the student lives. This major problem in first defining and them implementing the concept of "least restrictive" has been open to interpretation. Without question, it applies to the physical setting, i.e., the regular class is preferable to the special class. It would also apply to distance, i.e., children must attend the school they would attend if nonhandicapped unless the individual education plan specifies another arrangement. Duration should also be considered. One year in a specific room, such as a resource room, for half days might be more restrictive than one month in a self-contained, full day special class.

One of the criterion used in determining whether or not a

particular program is appropriate for a specific child is the concept of "least restrictive alternative." The principle of least restrictiveness in essence represents a large philosophical position. Educationally, it is based on the premise that all students, handicapped and nonhandicapped, should be educated in a system that does not restrict their interaction with their peers nor employ unusual instructional arrangements unless specifically stated in their individual program plan (IEP). In essence it calls for a school pattern that closely reflects the pattern that nonhandicapped students must follow as they go through their school years.

Continual references concerning least restrictiveness are made when discussing the term *mainstreaming,* and mainstreaming is often viewed as being synonymous with least restrictive environments in the public schools. Mainstreaming refers to the integration of eligible, exceptional students with normal peers based on their individual educational plan. It requires clarification of responsibility among regular, special education, administrative, instructional, and support personnel for implementation.

While legal authorities and educators will continue to argue over the definition of least restrictiveness, one fact becomes clear. It is essential that the handicapped student be placed in the last restrictive environment only when the knowledge of that placement leads to the belief that there is a high probability that the student will not only do well but that the placement has been modified to remediate any academic and/or interpersonal performance related deficits. Without this assurance, it is presumptuous to assume that one class setting is less restrictive than another, especially when there exists a tremendous lack of research data to support either position.

Full Services

The term "free appropriate public education" has been interpreted as meaning special education and all related services that would be required to implement the individual education program of a handicapped child. When related services are not available, it becomes obvious that the individual education plan cannot be fully implemented. According to the definition of *related services* found in Public Law 94-142, they would include the following:

1. auditology
2. counseling services

3. early identification
4. medical services (diagnostic only)
5. occupational therapy
6. parent counseling and training
7. physical therapy
8. psychological services
9. recreation
10. school health services
11. social work services in school
12. speech pathology
13. transportation

While it is clear that many handicapped individuals will not need all of these services, it is important to stress that when a service is needed and is not made available it is a denial of access to an appropriate program. Also, if the services offered are inadequate, i.e., the duration of time is less than what was requested or the amount of days requiring therapy or other related services are not commensurate with that outlined in the Individual Education Program (IEP), it is again a denial of access to an appropriate program.

Summary

The expansion of services for the handicapped over the last decade is due, in large part, to increased federal legislation. Much of the legislation for the handicapped was passed between 1951 and 1975 and provides funds to train personnel in all areas of disability and to support research and demonstration grants to explore problems relating to the education of exceptional children.

In 1965, the Elementary and Secondary Education Act (ESEA) became law, thus including the handicapped in the general education provisions of the federal government. Public Law 89-750, the ESEA Title VI Amendments of 1966, provided additional assistance in the education of the handicapped and established the Bureau of Education for the Handicapped (BEH), within the United States Office of Education, and the National Advisory Committee on the Handicapped.

The Developmental Disabilities Act of 1970 (PL 91-517) emphasized the federal government's efforts to provide a better life for the developmentally disabled, and it provided more efficient services by transferring power to those persons directly involved with providing assistance at state and local levels. In 1971, reflecting the movement toward specific legislation for the handicapped,

PL 91-230 repealed Title VI of the Elementary and Secondary Education Act, replacing it with The Education of the Handicapped Act (EHA). Civil rights legislation emerged shortly after with PL 93-112, the Rehabilitation Act of 1973, guaranteeing the rights of the handicapped in employment and in educational institutions that receive federal money.

It has been suggested that the forerunner of PL 94-142, the Education of the Handicapped Amendments of 1974 (PL 93-380), significantly increased the level of federal aid for the handicapped. It directed those states that had not already done so to move toward guaranteeing due process rights for handicapped children and their parents on the basis of a definite timetable. The Education Amendments of 1974 also made state funding conditional upon each state's submission of a plan that includes methods for identifying handicapped children currently receiving and not receiving service. Thus, PL 93-380 established the goal of providing full educational opportunity to all handicapped children. The passage of PL 94-142, the Education for All Handicapped Children Act of 1975, directed the separate and diverse commitments of state and federal governments to handicapped children, not as a matter of charity, but of public policy.

Today, unfortunately, the possibility exists that changing political climates may result in modifications on amendments to the Education of All Handicapped Children Acts (PL 94-142). The changes significantly may restrict the major goals and objectives of the Acts from being achieved.

PROCEDURAL SAFEGUARDS FOR THE HANDICAPPED

Public Law 94-142 and Section 504 of the 1973 Vocational Rehabilitation Act provides substantial legal safeguards for parents of handicapped children. The following are examples of these safeguards.

Due Process

Basically, there are three major elements of procedural due process: (1) the right to adequate notice; (2) the opportunity to be heard; and (3) the right to an impartial decision based on the facts presented. Simply stated this means that the parents have the right to know what action the school is contemplating with regard to the identification, evaluation, and placement of their handicapped child. When the parents feel they are not in agreement with some of these decisions, they may present evidence to contradict the school's recommendations and they may voice their own proposals. Unfortunately, the time it takes to arbitrate specific problems or grievances often frustrates the handicapped student's parents.

There are numerous rights of which a parent or individual advocating for a handicapped child is able to utilize during the due process procedure. These including the right to:

1. Obtain an independent evaluation
2. Examine all school records
3. Determine whether the hearing will be closed or open
4. Be represented by counsel at a hearing
5. Bring the student to the hearing
6. Keep the student in his or her current educational placement until all due process hearing appeals have been completed
7. Written notification about the hearing
8. Present evidence and testimony during the hearing
9. Prohibit information or evidence being presented which has not been disclosed 5 days before the hearing
10. Cross-examine and challenge testimony and evidence presented at a hearing
11. Receive a verbatim transcript (usually an audiotape) at reasonable cost
12. Appeal the decision of the hearing officer or hearing panel

The Individual Education Program (IEP)

Use of the IEP encourages handicapped children to be viewed more as individuals than as stereotyped members of a handicapped group. Accountability, in terms of achieving goals in specific periods of time, also becomes clearer.

Parent involvement, which has all too often been ignored or left to phone calls is also encouraged as part of the IEP process. Without this involvement, specific programs will not reflect parental concerns. Additionally, the IEP is a written document; therefore, it can be readily accessed and updated. The IEP, by its very nature, also encouraged participation on the handicapped student in regular education programs, hence fostering the mainstreaming philosophy of educating handicapped children with their non-handicapped peers. Lastly, the interdisciplinary nature of the evaluation process allows the student's educational program to be developed by a team rather than by a specific individual who may be unaware of the student's specific needs.

Record Keeping

Up until recently, parents were frustrated by their inability to have access to their child's school records. Traditionally these records were confidential and thus restricted from parental view. When they did review their child's records, some parents became upset over anecdotal notes and diagnostic information that was littered with unclear, or inaccurate jargon. When parents disagreed with its accuracy of what was contained within their child's record, they often did not know or were not apprised of the recourse or process they needed to follow for amending information.

Today, however, under The Family Educational Rights and Privacy Act (FERPA), often referred to as the *Buckley Amendment,* parents have the right to inspect and review any records relating to their children which are collected, maintained, or used by the school system for identification, evaluation, and placement of children in special education programs. Educational records, as defined by the regulations of the Buckley Amendment, are documents directly related to a student and maintained by an educational agency or institution or by a party acting for the agency or institution. Because the definition of an educational record is so complex, it is important that the parent or parent–teacher advocate understands that educational records are not documents related solely to education. For example, if a local education agency receives reports of a psychological evaluation from a community health center and maintains this report in its records, then the reports would be accessible to parents despite the fact that they may be stamped with the word "confidential."

Accessible records refer to those kept anywhere within a public school system. They do not refer only to those kept in a central cumulative file. In essence, records are accessible no matter where the local education agency keeps them.

Educational records relate not only to documents maintained by the system but to records maintained by other agencies who have performed services for the school system. For example, private evaluations performed at a clinic may very well be medically related, but if they are used to determine placement of a child, then they become part of the educational record of the student.

The parents also have a right to ask the school to provide a list of the types and locations of records kept on their child. For years parents who asked to see the record of a child were often shown incomplete information. Schools often had more than one file on a child as support personnel tended to keep their own records in separate locations. Until recently, parents were surprised to see the type of information that was kept on their child. Obviously, this led to a great amount of misunderstanding, frustrations, and distrust as the parent began to feel that information was being withheld from them.

When parents request records the school must comply without unreasonable delay and usually within 45 days. If a critical meeting has been called before this time, such as an IEP meeting or a hearing, the records must be made available before such a meeting takes place. After examining the records, the parents have the right to receive explanations and interpretations of their contents. They also have the right to make copies of the information. While there is no fee for searching out the requested information or retrieving it, there is a fee for duplicating information as long as the charge is not excessive or prohibitive. At this time no standard for what constitutes a fair cost per page has been determined.

It should be mentioned that some schools are reluctant to have parents view records for fear they will misunderstand or misinterpret some of the information. In some instances this is a valid assumption, since many handicapped individuals have complex records that require someone to interpret the terminology as well as the information regarding therapeutic intervention. The school should provide a staff member who will explain the information in a non-intimidating fashion. In some situations it is best to let the parents review the file in private and to list their questions or answers immediately after the review.

Parents who review records may find information that violates the right of privacy of the child or of themselves. Until now they have had very little recourse in which to amend this information. It is important to remember that while the parent does have the right to amend information in a record, it is still up to the school to decide, in a reasonable period of time, whether they will grant this request. If the school officials decide they cannot amend the record, they must notify the parents, explain them their rights, and bring the matter to a hearing on this issue. This specific hearing is not an "impartial due process hearing" since its procedures are governed by provisions of The Family Education Rights and Privacy Act. The parents must be given notice in advance of the hearing's place, date, and time so that they can present evidence and be assisted or represented by an attorney or other individuals of their choice. If the school officials decide not to amend the record, they must notify the parents of their right to place in the records a statement commenting on why they disagree with the school's information. This statement is attached to the record and must be maintained in the child's permanent record as long as it remains contested. Any dissenting view expressed by a parent must be shared with anyone reviewing the child's folder for information or educational decision-making purposes.

Confidentiality

Any disclosure of records that has personally identifiable information to anyone other than the parents or a designated representative must be closely monitored and controlled. The school must keep a list of employees who are authorized to see the records when it is determined by the school system they have legitimate educational interests. This list must be available to the public and other employees who do not fit under the rubric of school staff. The school system must always obtain parental consent before disclosing any information about a child's record. In addition to the school system, public and private agencies receiving records should maintain a list of all persons outside their organizations to whom access has been granted, including name, date, and purpose of the person authorized to use the records; also, those persons authorized to receive information may not redisclose it to any other parties without further parental consent. It has also been recommended that one official at each school or agency be placed in charge of ensuring confidentiality. The use of blanket permissions for disclosure that are usually signed when a child enters a program are often invalid because the parent at that time would not know what records would be disclosed at a future date.

An exception to parental consent does occur during health emergencies. When an emergency arises that is a serious threat to the health or safety of the child, specific information may be required to meet the emergency. At that time, specific personally identifiable information may be disclosed, but after the disclosure the parents must be kept informed as to what was released and to the party to whom the information was given.

Schools may destroy outdated diagnostic and anecdotal information when new information is received, such as after repeated evaluations of the child. The school should inform the parents of their desire to destroy outdated records that are no longer needed for educational planning. If the school and parents no longer need or want the information, it must be destroyed. The school may keep as part of a permanent record, however, the student's name, address, phone number, grades, classes attended, grade level completed, attendance record, and year completed.

Hearing Procedures

Under the present system of federal and most state laws any disagreement between the parents and the local education agency or school system regarding evaluation, identification, or educational placement of the child may be brought to a "due process hearing." Simply stated, *due process* means *fair procedure*. Under the law, schools must use fair procedures in all matters regarding parents, surrogate parents, and guardians as well as with students. Due process has long been one of the most important constitutional rights of parents and students.

While many states may have rules and regulations regarding hearing that are slightly different, the majority of the states conform to specific guidelines. For example, hearings must be convened no later than 45 days after there is a receipt of a written request for the hearing. It also must be conducted at a place and time that are reasonably convenient and mutually agreed upon by the parents, child, and the local education agency.

Parents also have the right to be notified in writing about the decision reached as a result of the local hearing. In some states the decision must be rendered within a specific number of days, that is 5 days, and written notification of the decision must be made to the parents within an additional 5 days. Most importantly, if the parents are still dissatisfied by the findings and the ultimate decision, they may appeal this decision within a specific number of days, that is, 30 days, to their state department of education. It is then incumbent upon their state department of education to conduct an impartial review of the hearing again within a specific numbers of days (30 days) of receipt of a written appeal. The state department using a panel then conducts a similar type of hearing and arrives at its own independent decision.

If parents still do not agree with the decision rendered by the State Department of Education they have the right to take civil action in their district court.

Impartial Hearing Officer

The law, even before recent federal legislation for the handicapped, has insisted upon impartiality in making administrative decisions. Traditionally, schools followed a simple model when problems materialized. The process typically consisted of having complaints first reviewed by the principal or administrator(s) of the school. If no solution could be reached, the complaints were usually brought to the attention of the area coordinator or superintendent of schools. If it could not be resolved there, a hearing was then convened before the school board. Today, however, recent federal legislation requires a somewhat different procedure for handicapped students. A parent now has the ability to select or utilize the services of an impartial hearing officer who is not an employee of the school system. Typcally, problems that cannot be resolved by the local school, region, or director or supervisor of special education for the local school district should be referred by the parent for an impartial hearing.

States must also have specific ways of determining the criteria for selecting a hearing officer in the most impartial way. For example, the hearing officer in some states is selected on a rotating basis from a list that has been developed from qualified individuals who have been certified to act in this capacity. Furthermore, a hearing officer in most states cannot be someone who is employed by the agency responsible for the child's education or care. Information concerning the impartial hearing officer's background can be made available to the parents for their review as well as for review by their legal counsel or advocate.

Parents and/or guardians also have the right to legal advice or counsel and may be accompanied to the hearing by this counsel. They also may be accompanied by individuals who have specific knowledge or training with respect to the problem of their child (i.e., reading teacher, teacher of the severely and profoundly handicapped, speech pathologist, pediatrician, and related therapy personnel).

During the hearing procedure parents either by themselves or with the help of their counsel have the right to present evidence and to question witnesses. They also have the right to compel the attendance of any witness who may have special knowledge or training about the problems of their specific child. Parents, as well as the local or state education agency, have the right to prohibit the introduction of evidence which has not been disclosed to them during a prior agreed upon time. This usually has been for 5 days and in many states is known as the "Five Day Rule." When appropriate, the child has the right to be present.

Additionally, the parents decide whether the hearing should be open or closed to the public. Parents also have a right to an account of the hearing. This has created some confusion in that the account has often been viewed as being a transcript of the proceedings. Unfortunately, due to the prohibitive cost of most transcripts many school systems will provide an audiotape to the parents at a minimum or no cost rather than actual typed transcript.

Finally, a child must remain in his present educational placement until all hearing procedures are completed. In this way the child cannot be harmed by hastily made decisions.

Tests and Evaluation

One important component of recent educational legislation is the area describing independent evaluations. Often parents have brought their child, without prior knowledge of the school, to an independent evaluator and have sent the bill for these services to the local school system, which has often resulted in the development of an adversary relationship between parents and school officials.

While parents can obtain a private evaluation from a qualified examiner that is not employed by the school system, the billing procedure needs to be carefully understood. For example, if a school can prove its original assessment was appropriate during an impartial due process hearing, it does not have to pay the cost of the independent evaluation. If, however, the evaluation provides significantly new information, which also results in additional findings in the specific hearing, the school may be asked to pay the bill. The independent evaluation in any circumstance becomes part of the record and must be considered in any educational decision about the student.

There are specific recommendations that may prove helpful to parents who undertake evaluations from the private sector:

1. Be sure that the evaluation is comprehensive and consists of more than one single test aimed at determining a cognitive level or I.Q. score.
2. A complete physical examination should be included as a secondary form of evaluation. Often, children with sensory impairments are significantly penalized on tests of cognition.
3. Discuss with the evaluator your observations of your child's behavior as well as his or her strengths and weaknesses.
4. Discuss with the evaluator the specific tests to be given and the reasons for their selection. It is also important to remember that your permission must be given before your child can be evaluated.

Most importantly, it is the equal responsibility of both professionals and parents to insist that the results of testing and evaluation be explained in clear, jargon-free terms. School and clinical evaluations esoterically written do little in terms of defining or explaining a child's educational strengths or weaknesses and serve little purpose in the development of a handicapped student's educational program.

REFERENCES

Brown *vs* Board of Education, 347. U.S. 483, (1954).
Code of Federal Regulations, U.S. Government Printing Office, Washington, D.C.
Federal Register, U.S. Government Printing Office, Washington, D.C.
Mills *vs* Board of Education, 348, F. Supp. 866 (D.D.C. 1972).
Pennsylvania Association for Retarded Children *vs* Commonwealth of Pennsylvania, 334 F. Supp. 1257 (E.D.P.A. 1971)
Public Law 89-10, Elementary and Secondary Education Act, (ESEA) 1965.
Public Law 89-750, Elementary and Secondary Education Act, (ESEA) Title VI Amendments, 1966.

Public Law 91-230, Education of the Handicapped Act, 1971.
Public Law 91-517, Developmental Disabilities Act of 1970.
Public Law 93-112, The Rehabilitation Act of 1973, Section 504, 29. U.S.C., 794, 1973.
Public Law 93-380, The Education Amendments of 1974, S. Rep. NO. 94-168., 1974.
Public Law 94-103, Developmentally Disabled Assistance and Bill of Rights Act, 45 CFR 1385, 1977.
Public Law 94-142, Education of Handicapped Children, Implementation of Part B of the Education of the Handicapped Act, Aug., 1977.
The Family Educational Rights and Privacy Act (FERPA), 20, U.S.C., 1232g, 1976.

SUGGESTED READINGS

Abeson, A., & Weintraub, F. Understanding the individualized education program. In S. Torres (ed.), *A primer on individualized education programs for handicapped children*. Reston, Virginia: The Foundation for Exceptional Children, 1977.

Agard, J., & Hoff, M. The ABT special teens and parents study of PL 94-142's Impact. Cambridge, Massachusetts: ABT Associates, 1979.

Ballard-Campbell, M. (ed.). Bureaucracy, law, and litigation. *Exceptional Education Quarterly*, 1981, *2* 1–93.

Bensky, J. M., Shaw, S. F., Gouse, A. S., Bates, H., et al. Public law 94-142 and stress: A problem for educators. *Exceptional Children* 1980, *47*, 24–29.

Biklen, D., & Bogdan, R. Handicappism in america. In B. Blatt, D. Bogdan, & R. Biklen, (eds). *An alternative textbook in special education*. Denver: Love Publishing Company, 1977.

Blaschke, C. Case study of the implementation of PL 94-142 (Final Report). Washington, D.C. Education Turnkey Systems, 1979.

Budoff, M. Engendering change in special education practices. *Harvard Educational Review*, 1975, *45*, 507–526.

Budoff, M., & Orenstein. *Due process in special education: The hearings process*. Cambridge, Massachusettes: Ware Press, 1981.

Bureau of Education for the Handicapped (DHEW). *Progress towards a free appropriate public education*. Washington, D.C.: Government Printing Office, 1980.

Burgdorf, R. *The legal rights of handicapped persons*. Baltimore: Brookes Publishing Company, 1980.

Cronin, J. Testimony regarding PL 94-142 on behalf of CCSSO and

NASDSE before select education/education and labor committee. Washington, D.C., 1979.

Friedman, R. *The rights of mentally retarded persons.* New York: Avon, 1976.

Haavik, S. F., & Menninger, K. *Sexuality, law and the developmentally disabled.* Baltimore: Brookes Publishing Company, 1981.

Henderson, R. A., & Hage, R. E. Economic implications of public education of the handicapped. *Journal of Research and Development in Education,* 1979, *12,* 71–79.

Higgins, S. T., & Barresi, J. The changing focus of public policy. *Exceptional Children,* 1979, *45,* 270–277.

Husk, S. B. Testimony regarding PL 94-142 on behalf of the council of greater city councils before select education/education and labor Committee. Washington, D.C., 1979.

Kaufman, M. J., Gottlieb, J. Agard, J., & Kukic, M.D. Mainstreaming: Toward an explication of the construct. In E. L. Meyen, G. A. Vergason, & R. J. Whelan (eds.), *Alternatives for teaching exceptional children.* Denver: Love Publishing Company, 1975.

Kotin, L., & Eager, N. B. *Due process in special education: A legal analysis.* Cambridge, Massachusettes: Research Institute for Educational Problems, 1977.

Lewis, L. *Project IEP: Washington State Report.* Arlington, Virginia: Nero and Associates, 1977.

14

Future Perspectives

TEACHER EDUCATION

One of the major barriers to implementing a program for severely disabled readers is the difficulty in obtaining qualified teachers. Many neophyte teachers from teacher training colleges do not understand the concepts and basic skills necessary for teaching in a successful remedial reading and learning disabilities program. The argument as to whether to emphasize subject matter courses or professional techniques courses has been waged for some time. The subject matter proponents appear to be in the ascendency. Local universities offer the most minimal undergraduate training in approaches to the teaching of reading. In fact, a secondary teacher of English or language arts can be graduated from many teacher training schools in the country and never have taken a course in the teaching of reading. The average primary teacher may be required to take one course in the teaching of reading or language arts.

To complicate matters, a large number of certified teachers never have had a college course in the teaching of reading, and many who have had such a course do not appear to really understand the basic language arts concepts. The situation becomes of greater concern when we realize that we are teaching reading by many different methods and that local schools change these methods from year to year. In addition, the schools often have not agreed upon one systematic sequence of skills. This lack of an organized and accepted sequence of skills for all children and the switching from one pedagogical procedure or material to another causes innumerable problems for our inexperienced and even experienced teachers.

The problem is much greater in the area of special education. Few colleges even recognize the condition of learning disabilities nor do they offer courses in the area at the undergraduate or graduate level.

School personnel now must view themselves as part of a human service delivery system rather than just a school system. New linkages must be developed between these agencies and new systems of training to bring about better collaboration among all the personnel participating in the human service delivery system.

In his article, "Public Law 94-142: A Matter of Human Rights" (1978), Dean Corrigan of the University of Maryland notes:

> The implications of placing the handicapped children in regular classrooms are enormous, not the least of which is that all educators—regular classroom teachers, counselors, administrators and other support personnel—must now be educated to work with persons with handicaps. Thus a change is called for in the roles of all educational personnel.
>
> (Corrigan, 1978, p. 18)

The ultimate goal is to extend the capacity of regular education personnel (teachers, administrators, and associated personnel) to accommodate a broad range of individual differences among students in order to prevent learning failure. The aggregate program adjustment required to meet these goals demands some fundamental changes in the professional preparation of teachers.

At present, general education, special education, early childhood education, speech and language development, psychology, and even reading methods usually are taught in separate departments or, perhaps at times, in different colleges within a university. Very few undergraduate or graduate students have an opportunity to be knowledgeable or even acquainted with the content of disciplines other than those included in their major field of study.

The curriculum of institutions of higher education should provide multidisciplinary training for all students. Every skilled teacher should be able to recognize possible learning difficulties and be knowledgeable about early preventive measures as well as prescriptive teaching methods necessary to overcome learning difficulties.

If educators cannot change the requirements or philosophies of the teacher training institutions, then the local school system must provide an ongoing program of inservice education and curriculum development. In other words, schools will not only need to teach children but also teach teachers.

Most present inservice programs consist of releasing teachers from their direct teaching responsibilities for 5 or 6 days during the school year. This approach has not effectively trained teachers in the area of the learning disabled. One sees a great deal of enthusiasm and interest generated but very little change or impact in the classroom. Theoretically, staff can be trained during the summer, but a summer program would be difficult to implement, since most local units cannot afford massive inservice programs.

Teacher education inservice, so desperately needed, can be conducted effectively at the local school level during the school day. Many administrators reject this concept of "released time," since it takes considerable planning and organization. Also, if local systems are going to train their own teachers, they must find instructors who understand the uniqueness of the learning disabled child and the unusual way in which he or she learns the language.

MEDICAL–EDUCATION COMMUNICATION

Educational problems as well as health services are a direct concern of the medical profession.

The involvement of medicine in the field of education has occurred due to a growing consensus of opinion that a substantial number of cases of reading failure do not result simply from poor teaching, absence of social and cultural opportunities, or insufficient motivation, but that they may be aggravated by specific defects in the central nervous system that cause perceptual difficulties.

Historically, communication between medically oriented diagnostic and evaluation institutions, and educational agencies has been notoriously poor: often the failure in communication occurs because written reports contain concepts and language foreign to the professional understandings of the educator and physician; secondly, the reports frequently do not reflect the reality of the educational or vocational placement of the client; and thirdly, the educational personnel often expect more than the medically oriented institution can or should provide. This lack of communication and interdisciplinary cooperation is becoming a serious deterrent to the successful implementation of Public Law 94-142.

A coordinate multidiscipline approach to the management and education of exceptional children and youth should be developed between medical and educational agencies concerned with the disabled. The objective of the interdisciplinary program would be to prepare educational personnel to work as case managers for educational services to exceptional children. Graduates of the program would be proficient in:

- Performing the appropriate evaluation in their specialty areas
- Participating in interdisciplinary evaluations and consultations
- Coordinating interdisciplinary evaluations and consultations
- Serving as translators between the interdisciplinary evaluation personnel and the instructional and remediation personnel
- Supervising the implementation of the instructional program
- Communicating to the interdisciplinary evaluation personnel the results of the diagnosis and the effectiveness of the instruction and the remediation program

VISUAL FACTORS AND THE
READING/LEARNING DISABLED CHILD

The field of learning disabilities has grown rapidly during the past 15 years. Numerous disciplines have become involved in the diagnosis and remediation of reading/learning disabilities in children, and many philosophies and treatment techniques have been espoused in the process. Perceptual development and training gained early attention of special educators, reading specialists, psychologists, optometrists, and others during this time.

Developmental vision optometrists feel that learning in general, and reading in particular, are primary visual perception tasks. The American Association of Ophthalmology and the American Academy of Pediatrics (1973), however, state that there is no peripheral eye defect that produces dyslexia and associated learning disabilities.

The wide variety of opinion by vision specialists has resulted in great confusion among parents and teachers. More important, this confusion has, in many cases, delayed the appropriate diagnosis and remediation of the disabled child.

The disciplines must come to some agreement if professionals are going to communicate and cooperate in interdisciplinary conferences and instructional programs.

COMPUTER-MANAGED INSTRUCTION FOR
READING/LEARNING DISABLED CHILDREN

Computer-managed instruction is fast becoming a priority for all teachers and students. Nationwide, about 50 percent of school districts provide students access to one computer, and 25 percent of all public schools have a computer available for students.

There is no greater support and enthusiasm for this new technology than in the field of special education. Nowhere are the benefits of learning with personal computers more dramatic than with the handicapped whose physical, cognitive, perceptual, or learning limitations have been a barrier to education and a productive life. At the other end of the continuum, computer-assisted instruction is just as essential for gifted and talented students.

Watkins & Webb (1981) have detailed some major impediments to the widespread adoption of microcomputers in education.*

1. Articles dealing with computer-assisted instruction have often been based upon speculation and conjecture rather than upon sound empirical research. Even when data were reported, serious methodological flaws often threatened both internal and external validity of results.
2. There is a scarcity of good educational software. Programmers of commercial software products for computers may not recognize GIGO, but many educators using computers do. An acronym, it means "garbage in and garbage out." "The computer," said one computer expert, "Has been embarrassed by the things it has been asked to do."
3. Training educational personnel to use computers is very difficult, especially when some think of themselves as technologically deficient. If teachers are predisposed to being afraid of computers, they are not going to welcome them into the classroom.

---

*Copyright 1981 by Educational Computer, P.O. Box 535, Cupertino, California 95015. Sample issue $3.00, 6-issue subscription $15.00. Reprinted with permission.

4. A final and often overlooked barrier to the acceptance and widespread diffusion of technological innovations, including microcomputers, lies in the complex human dynamics of schools. A teacher survey found about half of the teachers not interested in computer training. The remarks of a teacher are even more graphically illustrative of this problem. "Every ten years or so there's something new in educational technology that's touted as a panacea," she stated. "A few years back it was instructional television and machine learning; now it's microcomputers. Once the newness of the gadget wears off, we return to the basic need for teacher–student interaction." It is apparent from such survey and interview results that potent human dynamic factors must be considered and overcome before widespread adoption of microcomputers in education occurs.

If educators are to understand how computers can help the exceptional child, specialists from several fields, including engineers, educators, physicians, psychologists, and the intended handicapped users themselves must share their collective knowledge and experience. This interdisciplinary approach is vital if an effective and practical use of computer technology to aid the exceptional child is to be achieved.

SELF-ESTEEM AND THE LEARNING DISABLED CHILD

Research with nonhandicapped children of school age overwhelmingly supports a relationship between self-esteem and academic performance. It is assumed that the learning disabled youngster is subject to the same factors in the development of self-concept as the normal child. There may be certain factors unique to the handicapping condition, in addition to the disability itself, which influence self-concept.

These assumptions focus on the belief that learning disabled children have poorer attitudes toward themselves and, as a result, achieve less and exhibit more behavior problems in the classroom. The literature reports that behavior disorders are related to learning disability; however, the influence of self-esteem in relation to behavior disorders has not been fully addressed.

Research is needed to examine the relationship between self-esteem and achievement motivation in learning disabled children by investigating the following questions:

1. Do learning disabled children have low self-esteem?
2. Is there a subgroup of learning disabled children who can profit from self-esteem remediation in conjunction with academic remediation?
3. How is self-esteem "remediation" best accomplished?

VOCATIONAL EDUCATION FOR THE SEVERE READING DISABLED

With the passage of Public Law 94-142, it has become critical that handicapped students' Individual Education Programs (IEPs) include a prevocational or vocational education component. Traditional efforts to develop a vocational battery have tended to focus upon the needs of regular classroom students and not the handicapped.

Instruments currently in use to describe student vocational behaviors and performances have not been specifically adapted for use with severe reading disabled populations, resulting in the absence of vocational information in many handicapped students' educational plans.

The use of appropriate vocational evaluation instruments has also undergone criticism, in that their administration has not always been responsive to Public Law 94-142's mandate which ensures the evaluation of handicapped students in their native languages and through appropriate modes of communication. Research in the vocational area is just beginning and will need to be expanded to all populations of handicapped individuals.

RESEARCH AND EVALUATION

Research has emphasized the complexities of the problem rather than the solutions. Since there are few controlled studies for remediation, educators and others have turned to panaceas and pseudoscientific methods that are usually justified by articles that appear in popular magazines rather than in professional journals.

Instead of expounding methods of treatment based on the enthusiasm of vested interests, concerned professionals should adopt as guidelines for educational programs controlled basic research that is unbiased and applicable to large groups of students rather than a small population.

In almost all new innovative educational activities there is great difficulty in convincing people of the need for longitudinal experimental programs in which the approaches and techniques are kept pure for the length of the study. Strong efforts must be made to resist contamination with personal interpretations and biases.

Remediation programs, if they are successful, will be at best a slow process and only the teacher and other persons who are directly involved will see the slow changes in behavior of the students. These behavioral changes are difficult to measure objectively. Consequently, the evaluation of such programs should include input from individuals directly involved.

It is important that effective longitudinal research be carried on somewhere in the country because too often local school systems will insist on supportive research before starting a new program. Studies must be longitudinal because the research just does not exist to show the amount of remission, the most effective teaching procedures, the optimum starting grade level, and the amount and length of therapy.

REFERENCES

Corrigan, D. Public law 94-142: A matter of human rights. In J. Grosenick, & M. Reynolds (eds.): *A call for change in schools and colleges of education: Renegotiating roles for mainstreaming.* Reston, VA: Council for Exceptional Children, 1978, pp. 17–29.

Education USA. Washington, D. C.: National School Public Relations Association (newsletter), *23:* February 2, 1981.

The eye and learning disabilities. Joint organizational statement. Washington, D.C.: The Executive Committee and Council of the American Academy of Pediatrics, the American Academy of Ophthalmology and Otolaryngology, and the American Association of Ophthalmology, 1973.

Watkins, M., & Webb, C. Computer assisted instruction with learning disabled students. *Educational Computer Magazine,* Sept–Oct., 1981, 24–27.

Glossary

Accommodative Convergence: As part of the near reflex, there is convergence of the visual axes associated with accommodation. A fairly consistent increment of accommodative convergence (AC) occurs for each diopter of accommodation (A) giving the accommodative convergence/accommodation ratio (AC/A). Abnormalities of this ratio are common and are important in causing strabismus. If there is an abnormally high accommodative convergence/ accommodation ratio, the excess convergence tends to produce estotropia during accommodation or near targets. If there is an abnormally low accommodative convergence/accommodation ratio, the eyes will tend to be exotropic when the individual looks at near target.

Act: A law passed by a legislature; statute.

Adaptive Teaching: Those methods, materials, and management techniques selected to circumvent a learning disabled student's specific areas of disabilities and maximize areas of abilities. Adaptive teaching is synonymous with compensatory teaching, i.e., helping the student compensate for the disabilities.

This glossary consists of definitions of terms as used within the context of this book.

Alexia: A label used to designate a cerebral disorder characterized by the inability to read. "Word blindness" is another term used in this connection.

Amicus Curiae: "Friend of the court." This term refers to a third party—a person or organization — who, while having no direct legal interest in the outcome of a lawsuit, submits briefs and, on occasion, evidence to a court in support of a position.

Amblyopia: A unilateral or bilateral loss of corrected central visual acuity without a visible organic lesion commensurate with this loss. Incidence is about 2 to 2½ percent in the general population. Characteristics are eccentric fixation and crowding phenomenon. The two types of amblyopia are strabismic amblyopia and anisometropic amblyopia.

Appeal: An application to a higher court to reverse, modify, or change the ruling of a lower court. The United States Supreme Court is the highest court of appeals in the country.

Architectural Barriers: Structural and physical obstructions that exclude or discriminate against handicapped people, i.e., steps, curbs, inaccessible bathrooms, elevators, phone booths, etc.

ARD Committee: Admission, Review, and Dismissal Committee (required by some states, but not required by federal law) comprised of individuals familiar with the child's current level of functioning (i.e., direct services deliverers, health department personnel, and special educators). The ARD Committee refers for placement and reviews the individual educational program of every handicapped child on a yearly basis.

Assessment: Extensive procedure given to all children who have been identified through screening as potentially in need of special education programs.

Auditory Discrimination: The ability to discriminate between sounds of different characteristic frequencies. It may invoke differentiating tone, rhythm, volume, or direction of sound.

Background of Information: The accumulated experiences of the individual in terms of factual data, relationships among facts, etc.

Basal Reader Approach: The development of basic reading abilities and skills by means of a series of graded readers with a controlled vocabulary. It is usually used in a teacher-directed reading activity spelled out in an accompanying manual.

Bibliography: Use of reading as an approach to understanding of self and solution of personal problems.

Bill: A proposed statute, not yet law.

Board (or Local Board):   A county or city board of education.

Brief: A lawyer's written summary of the law and/or facts involved in a particular case.

Capacity Tests: Tests designed to measure the individual's mental endowment or capacity for learning. The intelligence quotient or mental age derived from such a test is the current functioning level and may be depressed, in terms of the innate capacity, by such factors as limitations of experience and emotional disturbances.

Central Dominance: The control of activities by the brain, with one hemisphere usually being considered consistently dominant over the other. Confusion in this control may be indicative of neurological damage. Measurement of central dominance is made through outward performance, but in situations that have not become familiar to the individual through practice.

Class Action: A lawsuit brought by one or more named persons on their own behalf and on behalf of all persons in similar circumstances. A court's ruling in a class action suit applies to all members of the "class."

Color Coding Approach: Another approach to solve the problems of the inconsistent orthography of the English language. It superimposes consistency upon standing English orthography by adding the dimension of color. The color coders superimpose a single, invariant color upon a given vowel sound in the printing of their materials regardless of the variety of ways in which that sound is normally represented in written form.

Common Law: The body of law derived from historical usage, as opposed to statutory (written) law.

Complaint: A formal legal document submitted to a court by one or more persons, alleging that their rights have been violated. A complaint specifies one or more causes of action, names those who have allegedly violated the rights, and demands that the defendents take certain corrective action.

Concept Burden of Materials: A measure of the meanings represented by the language in the reading materials. It should consider both the difficulty of the concepts (the experience needed to form them and the complexity of their organization) and the density of concepts (number of different concepts appearing in a given amount of material). This burden is a potent factor in determination of the difficulty level of the material.

Concepts: Two or more related experiences that fuse together to form a broader idea or understanding. They are always built basically from concrete (actual or direct) experiences. When vicarious experience is used, it in turn must be related back to concrete experiences for understanding, since a vicarious experience is seldom as reliable as a direct experience. In reading, concepts are used, rearranged, organized, and reorganized as the reader reads; they are *basic* to comprehension in reading.

Conclusions of Law: A judge's application of the law to the facts in a specific case.

Consent (Informed Consent):   An intelligent, knowing, and voluntary agreement by someone to a given activity or procedure. Three conditions must exist before informed consent can be given: (1) the person must be capable of understanding the circumstances and factors surrounding a particular consent decision: (2) information relevant to the decision must be forthrightly intelligibly provided to the person; and (3) the person must be free to give or withhold consent voluntarily.

Consent Agreement: A court-ratified and court-enforced agreement between the opposing parties to a suit resolving the consented issues. Reached after the initiation of a lawsuit, a consent agreement, because it is ratified by a court, carries the same weight as any other court order.

Constitutional Right: A right guaranteed by the United States Constitution or the constitution of the state in which a person resides. A federal constitutional right supersedes federal or state law.

Defendant: The party against whom a lawsuit is filed.

Developmental Teaching: As built into the regular methods and content of instruction of the school, it is used with the learning disabled student to achieve those goals of education for all students. Developmental teaching is defined as those materials, methods, and management techniques approved by the local education agency (LEA) that are usually successful with normally developing children. Necessary modifications to meet the unique needs of the learning disabled students may be provided.

Directed Reading Activity: A reading lesson based on basal-reader material. Provision is made for readiness, silent reading for survey purposes, vocabulary and comprehension development, silent or oral rereading, and follow-up.

Due Process: A right guaranteed under the Fifth and Fourteenth Amendments to the United States Constitution to have any law applied reasonably and with sufficient safeguards, such as hearings and notices to ensure that an individual is dealt with fairly. A due process hearing is held when there is disagreement between the parent and the educational agency (either local or state) as to the identification, evaluation and/or placement of a handicapped child into a special education program. Parents have the right to present evidence, to require the attendance of witnesses, to cross-examine witnesses, and to obtain independent assessments.

Early Identification: Programs provided by local education agencies for the preschool age child who may be in need of special education services.

Eclectic Approach: The "smorgasbord" technique in which the student is exposed to a combination of approaches and/or methods of reading instruction. This does not have to be classified as a "hit or miss" procedure. A skilled teacher using an effective diagnostic-prescriptive approach may effectively employ this technique.

Equal Protection: A right guaranteed by the Fourteenth Amendment. This clause of the U.S. Constitution states that all citizens are entitled to equal protection under the law, that is, to be free from discrimination in the exercise of rights except where the state demonstrates a rational basis or compelling interest for apparently unequal treatment.

Evaluation: An additional review of the child's program that occurs at least annually and is conducted to determine: (1) whether the child has achieved the goals set forth in his or her individualized education program (IEP), (2) whether the child has met the criteria which would indicate readiness to enter into a less restrictive/ intensive special education program, and (3) whether the program the child is in should be specifically modified so as to be more suitable for the child.

Evidence: Written documentation or oral evidence submitted to a court in support of the position of one of the opposing parties to a suit. A complex set of rules governs the admission of evidence in court.

Exceptional Child: One who deviates significantly from the norm. May be exceptional by virtue of unusually high or low intelligence, physical disabilities, etc.

Experience: (1) Direct — actual participation in an event or events from immediate sensory stimulation; (2) vicarious — substitute participation in an event or events (language, pictures, etc. may substitute for the actual ojbect or event).

Expressive Language: Abilitty to recall relevant words and sentences and to develop those ideas into a meaningful sequence for the motor act of speech.

Factual Question: A type of comprehension question that requires, as a response, information definitely stated in the reading material.

FAPE: Free Appropriate Public Education.

Fernald Approach: Teachers employing the Fernald Approach usually begin with a tracing step. At this stage the learner listens as the teacher writes the word. The learner observes the writing, says the word as he/she traces (continuing until he/she can write the word) and says it as he/she writes it. As the child progresses, he/she no longer needs the tracing, but otherwise follows the same type of procedure. Throughout the stages, words are learned as wholes, being pronounced naturally and in syllables as they are traced, studied, or written. This tracing technique is an attempt to achieve maximum stimulation for word learning.

FERPA: Family Education Rights and Privacy Act — also known as the Buckley Amendment — permits parents to examine and copy (at reasonable cost) any and all material in the child's permanent records.

Figurative Language: Use of words to convey a meaning other than their literal meaning.

Follow-Up: Activity designed to strengthen abilities that have been introduced in directed reading activity to provide needed practice of abilities, to broaden or deepen concepts, to provide additional experience with the area of content, to allow further related reading, and so on.

Frustration Level: The level at which the child "bogs down" because he/she is unable to comprehend what he/she is trying to read. At this level the child acquires undesirable habits and attitudes and becomes discouraged. (Achievement test score usually represents this level.)

Fusional Convergence: If the visual axes diverge from the object of regard, the brain will reduce this disparity error to zero by converging the eyes without changing their refractive state.

Generalizing: A process of determining the essential similarity in a group of individual ideas, discarding the differences between the individual ideas, and operating in terms of the similarity. On the verbal level, generalizing involves being able to state the common element: to provide a label for it. Requires moving from a group of ideas or objects to a broader one which includes the original group.

Gillingham Approach: In contrast to the Fernald analytical approach, the Gillingham is a synthesis procedure. The Gillingham technique advocates teaching the sounds of the letters and then building these letter sounds into words, like bricks into a wall. Many educators associate this method with the familiar "phonetic" or "sound" technique. The difference lies in the fact that the Gillingham approach is based on the close association of visual, auditory, and kinesthetic elements.

Guardian: An individual who has the legal authority to make decisions on behalf of another.

Handicapped Children: Those children who have been determined through appropriate assessment as having temporary or long-term special education needs arising from cognitive, emotional, or physical factors or any combination of factors.

Hearing Comprehension Level: The reading level at which the child is able to understand materials adequately when they are read to him or her. Comprehension should be at least 75 percent and the child should show oral vocabulary of a level commensurate with that used in the selection.

IHO: Impartial Hearing Officer. A person who is knowledgeable in the fields and areas significant to the review of the child's education.

Independent Reading Level: Is the book level at which a child can read independently with ease, enjoyment, and complete understanding, without evidence of tension. This is the level at which a child should do supplementary reading, such as unsupervised library reading for enjoyment or information.

IEP: Individualized Education Program. A written comprehensive outline for total special education services that describes the special education needs of the child and the services to be provided to meet those needs. It is developed in a collaborative meeting with the local education agency (LEA) representatives, parents, teachers, the student, when appropriate, and all other persons having direct responsibilities for the implementation of the IEP. The IEP must be developed before placement, approved by the admission, review, and dismissal (ARD) Committee, and signed by the parent.

Individualized Reading Approach: A planned approach in which students read independently (often in trade books) and are instructed by the teacher individually, in relation to the book being read, and in small groups, for skill development. Any method by which students are allowed to progress independently of the group is usually termed "individualized."

Inferential Question: A type of comprehension question that tests the ability to draw a specific conclusion from facts explicitly stated.

Initial Teaching Alphabet Approach: The ITA is an approach, not a method. It is one of several systems devised to attack the problem of phonemic multirepresentation by the English system of orthography. ITA's proposed solution is to make a *temporary* change in the orthography of the English language for beginning readers through the creation of a consistent phoneme–grapheme relationship.

Instructional Reading Level: Is the highest book level at which a pupil is able to read with success under the teacher's guidance. It is the level at which the teacher begins purposeful, teacher-directed reading (Basal reading level).

Intelligence Tests: Tests that are supposed to measure the individual's mental endowment or capacity for learning. Factors actually tapped by the tests are those which investigators have felt were the components of what is known as intelligence. The intelligence quotient or mental age derived from such a test is the current functioning level of intelligence and may be depressed, in terms of the innate capacity, by limitation of experience, emotional disturbances, organic factors, etc.

Jurisdiction: The authority of a court to hear and decide a suit.

Language Experience Approach: This approach has students who have participated in a common experience discuss that experience. Then the teacher dictates a short story about it (a few sentences) which the pupils, if they are capable, or the teacher writes down. The story then becomes the material used for teaching reading (including the mastery of a basic sight vocabulary). In some clinical situations this approach, coupled with the Fernald multisensory technique, has proven effective with many disabled readers.

Laterality: A general term used to cover patterns of dominance of the eye, foot, and/or hand.

LEA: Local Education Agency, also known as the LSS (Local School System). The LEA is responsible for providing the actual education children receive.

Linguistic Approach: The solution proposed by the present day descriptive linguists for the inconsistent orthography of the English language is one of delay. In brief, they advocate the presentation of words, which only represent regular or consistent relationships between sounds and printed symbols in the beginning stages of reading, with a delayed, gradual, and systematic introduction of irregular phoneme–grapheme correspondences.

LRE: Least Restrictive Environment. The educational setting that is considered educationally appropriate, to the maximum extent possible, for handicapped children.

Mechanical Aids/Computer Approach: The application of mechanical and electronic technology to aid the teaching of the communication skills has developed great support, enthusiasm, and anticipation in the education community. Since the 1940s, tachistoscopes and pacers have been widely used in speed reading programs. Presently, some schools use personal computers to help students with specific subjects, such as mathematics or reading, and to challenge high achievers.

Mills: The name of the lead plaintiff in *Mills vs. Board of Education of the District of Columbia,* a landmark class action right-to-education suit on behalf of children with disabilities. The Mills case established the rights of disabled children to a suitable publicly supported education and to due process in education and placement decisions. The basic principles of Mills and *PARC vs. Pennsylvania* were later incorporated into PL 94-142.

Memory Span: Refers to the number of items that can be recalled immediately after presentation. The phenomena of memory are often classified as fixation, retention, recall, and recognition.

Motion: A request to the court in the context of a specific case to take some action relating to the case.

Neurological: Of or related to the nervous system. Neurological problems are those arising from disease or of damage to the nervous system.

Nondiscriminatory Legislation: Nondiscrimination on the basis of handicap. Federal rules and regulations prohibiting discrimination against handicapped persons by any agency or organization that is assisted by Federal funds. The regulations call for: (1) a free appropriate education for all handicapped children, regardless of the nature or severity of the handicap; (2) positive employment and job opportunities; (3) the elimination of architectural barriers; (4) adaptive education at the college and postsecondary level; and (5) equal treatment of the handicapped by health, welfare, and social services agencies. These regulations apply to states, counties, cities, public and private schools, colleges, universities, hospitals, clinics, and numerous other recipients of federal funds thatt provide program and services.

Nonpublic Special Education School: Approved private special education facility where a child is placed when an appropriate program of spcial education and related services for the child is not available in the local education agency. These schools may be day or residential, and instate or out-of-state.

Nonpublic Tuition Assistance: In cases in which the local education agency (LEA) determines that it cannot provide the program needed for a given handicapped child, the LEA applies to the state for approval of (1) a specific placement, (2) funding of per pupil costs, (3) the program itself, and (4) the need of the child for the program.

Organic: Pertaining to internal organs. Organic involvement in reading disability means that the problem arises from or is complicated by disease or dysfunction within the body systems. (An organic-like case is one which has the functional characteristics of organicity but on a psychogenic basis rather than on a true organic basis.)

Parent Surrogate: A person who represents the child as his/her legal representative in the educational decision-making process when the child's own parents are unknown or unavailable.

Perception: Process by which the CNS organizes the sensory data.

Performance Test: A test composed of items that involve no manipulation of language, oral or visual, except for the interpretation and following of directions. Such test items are particularly essential when measuring the functional intelligence level of reading disability cases.

Peripheral Dominance: Handedness, eyedness, etc., and the relationships among them. Those factors of laterality that are observable in outward activities.

Persevervation: Persistance of previous responses in spite of their lack of application to the present situation. May be evidenced in repetition of words or in patterns of thought or action that previously satisfied a purpose different from the present one.

Petitioner: The party appealing a court's decision to a higher court. Synonym for appellant. Also sometimes used to identify the plaintiff in certain courts or types of cases.

PL 94-142:   Public Law 94-142. Federal legislation, also known as the Education of All Handicapped Children Act — a law governing provisions which are designed (1) to assure that all handicapped children have available to them a free, appropriate public education; (2) to assure that the rights of handicapped children and their parents are protected; (3) to assist states and localities to provide for the education of handicapped children; and (4) to assess and assure the effectiveness of efforts to educate such children.

Plaintiff: The party who brings a lawsuit, alleging a violation of rights.

Pleadings: The documents submitted to a court in the pretrial stage of litigation.

Position Maintenance System: This is not a movement system. Its function is to maintain an object of interest on the fovea or to maintain a specific gaze position. It is the most complex type of eye movement coordination and has its own micromovement system. It interacts with all other eye movement systems and is seriously disturbed when the patient's level of consciousness is depressed.

Precedent: A prior court decision in a relevant case, cited in the interpretation of a law or constitutional provision. A court may or may not accept a precedent as authoritative in interpreting the law in a specific case.

Preliminary Injunction: A temporary order to prevent a party from taking cartain actions pending the court's final decision.

Procedural Safeguards: Those state and federal rights guaranteed to a handicapped child and his/her parents relative to the acquisition of a free appropriate public education (FAPE). These include, but are not limited to, the right to see and copy records, the right to prior notice regarding a proposed program change, and the right to a due process hearing.

Programmed Reading Approach: In this approach there is a sequential presentation of bits of information in small steps or frames, each requiring a response on the part of the student. Answers are then revealed for immediate feedback. Students progress at their own rate, the teacher's role is to monitor progress and administer progress tests at specified intervals. For reading programs linguistically oriented material stressing phoneme-grapheme correspondences is usually used.

Protection and Advocacy Systam (P&A):   A state system to protect and advocate the rights of people with developmental disabilities (DD), as provided for by the DD Act. The DD Act requires states receiving federal DD money to establish a P&A system and provides for federal allotments to fund this system. Under the DD Act, the P&A system must be independent of any agency that provides services to persons with developmental disabilities, and it must have the authority to pursue legal, administrative, and other appropriate remedies.

Readability Level: An indication of the difficulty of reading material in terms of the grade level at which it is to be read. In many cases, the difficulty is measured by the vocabulary and the length and complexity of the sentences.

Readiness: A condition of adequacy in relation to all factors involved in the task to be performed.

Receptive Language: The interpretation of auditory stimuli and the extraction of meaning from words and sentences.

Related Educational Services: (1) Transportation and (2) developmental, corrective, and other supportive services that are required to assist a handicapped child in benefiting from education. These include speech pathology and audiology, psychological services, physical and occupational therapy, recreation, early identification and assessment of disabilities, counseling services, school health services, social work services in schools, parent counseling and training, and medical services for diagnostic or evaluation purposes.

Relief: The remedy to some legal wrong or violation of one's rights.

Remand: An order by a higher court returning a case to a lower court for further action consistent with the higher court's decision.

Remedial Teaching: Those methods, materials, and management techniques selected to ameliorate a learning disabled child's specific areas of disability identified through the assessment process and stated in the individual education program (IEP).

Respondent: Appellee. The winning party at the trial level in a case that has been appealed; the defendant in certain courts or cases.

Retinal Rivalry (Binocular Rivalry): The state that arises when corresponding areas of the two retinas are stimulated by nonfusable images (they may be antagonistic in color, contrast, or contour). A state of rapid alternation of parts of the stimulus ensues, and one or the other predominates in a given area at a given time.

Saccadic Movements: Require a sudden, strong pulse of force from the extraocular muscles in order to move the eye rapidly against the viscosity produced by the fatty tissue and fascia in which the globe lies. To abduct the eye in a saccade, there is a sudden great increase in lateral rectus activity to get the eye moving and, at the same time, a total inhibition of the medial rectus until the eye is again stabilized in the new gaze position. Velocity is nearly proportional to the size of saccade and can be $10°$/second to $600°$/second.

Saccadic System: Generates all fast eye movements, primarily refixation movements, to place an object of interest on the fovea or to move the eyes from one subject to another. An intact frontal cortex seems necessary to facilitate these movements.

Screening: Initial procedure for identifying problems that impede learning. It is provided to most kindergarten children and to those children who may be evidencing educational difficulties. Screening should include, but not be limited to: developmental information, previous assessments, visual, auditory, and motor functioning, and expressive and receptive language ability. Screening will be done in the child's primary language, if other than English.

SEA: State Education Agency, i.e., State Department of Education.

Selective Attention: Allows children to focus purposefully and for an appropriate length of time on incoming data that will lead to productive learning.

Shall/May: The term "shall" in a law, regulation, or court order is mandatory, while the term "may" is discretionary. The term "may" allows flexibility in a party's actions, including the flexibility not to act at all.

Sovereign Immunity: The legal doctrine that protects the state and federal governments from certain kinds of suits in certain courts on the general theory that the government ("sovereign") should be free to exercise its authority within reasonable limits. This immunity may be lost when the government exceeds its authority or acts in an unconstitutional manner. Recent laws and court decisions have greatly narrowed the concept of governmental immunity from suit.

Special Education: Public instruction provided at no cost to the parent, specifically designed to meet the unique needs of a handicapped child. This includes instruction provided in classrooms, homes, hospitals, or institutions.

Special Master: A person appointed by a court to monitor, implement, or supervise the implementation of the court's order or to provide reports to a court prior to a decision. Appointment of a special master is usually based on a defendant's presumed inability to implement a court's order.

State Board: The State Board of Education.

Statute: A law passed by a state or federal legislature; an act.

Stay: A court order postponing the enforcement of a court ruling pending future legal action, such as an appeal to a higher court.

Stereopsis: The sensation of relative depth and the ability to judge distance.

Stipulation: An agreement between parties in a lawsuit that certain facts are true.

Student Profile: A method of evaluating individual cases according to the interrelationships among test findings, educational history, parent interview, and observations for the purpose of making valid recommendations.

Study Skills: A term frequently used to cover comprehension abilities in the area of organization of ideas. Such abilities as getting main ideas annd supporting details, following various types of sequence, etc., are usually subsumed under "study skills." Application of these and related abilities (outlining, finding topic sentences, summarizing, etc.) are also included.

Summary Judgment: A judge's ruling on the law in a case where the judge holds that the facts are not in dispute.

Temporal-Sequential Organization: Development of time and sequence. Visual and auditory sequences affect short and intermediate memory.

Tonic Convergence: The position of the eyes in deep anesthesia is one of moderate exotropia. When the individual awakens, the eyes move into alignment by tonic convergence.

Tort: A civil wrong for which a private individual may recover money damages. False imprisonment and invasion of privacy are examples of torts.

VAKT: A word-learning techinque that makes use of visual, auditory, kinesthetic, and tactile stimulation. The child learns by tracing words, which he/she pronounces or hears pronounced as they are written for him/her, and so on. Words come from the child's own oral language background and are learned and written to satisfy present needs (see *Fernald* and *Gillingham Approaches*).

Verbal Test: A test composed of items that involve the manipulatuon of language in oral or written form. Certain intelligence tests employ both verbal and nonverbal or performance sections, thus providing opportunity for comparison of achievement on the two types.

Verdict: A judge's or jury's decision in favor of one of the parties in a lawsuit.

Versatility: Ability to vary the approach the reader uses to the reading material. The approach must be adjusted in terms of both the material and the purpose for which it is being read.

Visual Discrimination: The ability to see likenesses and differences between visual patterns. Involves discrimination of letter forms and word patterns, as well as the discrimination of gross forms.

Visual—Motor Coordination: Obtaining of data through vision and executing a motor movement (praxia), e.g., tying shoelaces or catching a ball.

Visual Perception: The phenomenon of understanding a stimulus that is received by the visual system and that results in cognition.

Visual—Spatial Orientation: The learning of spatial relationships by moving bodies and obtaining feedback from visual, kinesthetic, tactile and proprioceptive sensory pathways.

Index

Electroencephalogram (EEG),
  neurological disorders and,
  51–54
Electronystagmograph, 75–79
Elementary and Secondary
  Education Act of 1965, 127,
  169–170
  Title I, 128
Emotional instability, neurological
  disorders and, 44–45
Emotionally disturbed children,
  27–28
Emotional problems (emotional
  disturbances). *See also*
  Psychological disorders
  as defined in Public Law 94-142,
  165
  evaluation of, 30–31
Encephalitis, 42–43
Epilepsy, 48, 49, 52
Etiology of reading disabilities,
  7–8
Evaluation of learning disabilities.
  See also Psychological
  evaluation
  legal aspects of, 177–178
  remediation programs and,
  144–147
Eyedness, handedness and, 89
Eye glasses, 72
Eye movements (ocular motility),
  70–79
  in blind people, 79
  comprehension and, 77–79
  pursuit, 73–74
  reading and, 75–82
  saccadic, 72–73
  tests of, 71–72, 75
  vergences, 74
  vestibular, 74
Eyes. *See also* Vision
  anatomy and functioning of,
  69–70

dominance and controlling, 95
Eye tests, 71–72

Family Education Rights and
  Privacy Act (FERPA), 166,
  172–174
Family environment, psychiatric
  disorders and, 60, 66–67
Family history of reading disability,
  119
Far-sightedness (hyperopia), 72
Federal programs, coordination
  among, 127–131
Federal Register, 161
Federal regulations, 161
Fernald approach to reading
  instruction, 154–155
Fetal anoxia, 48, 49
Filtration technique, 79–81
"Five Day Rule," 177
Food additives, 112
Fourteenth Amendment, 161–162
"Free and appropriate education,"
  concept of, 167–169
Frostig Perceptual Tests, 85
Functional life skills, instruction in,
  150–151

General intelligence, 21–22
Genetics of reading disabilities,
  117–123
  chromosome aberrations,
  117–119
  evidence for genetic inheritance,
  118, 119
  familial history, 119
  pedigree analysis, 121
Geometric drawing, neurological
  disorders and difficulties in, 49,
  50
Gerstmann's syndrome, 92–93

a
b
c
d
e
f
g
h
i
8 2 j